# Current Clinical Strategies

## Psychiatry

**2008 Edition**

D1571551

*Rhoda K Hahn, MD*

*Lawrence J. Albers, MD*
Associate Clinical Professor
Department of Psychiatry and Human Behavior
University of California, Irvine, College of Medicine

*Christopher Reist, MD*
Professor and Vice Chairman
Department of Psychiatry and Human Behavior
University of California, Irvine, College of Medicine

*Current Clinical Strategies Publishing*

*www.ccspublishing.com/ccs*

Current Clinical Strategies Publishing
PO Box 1753
Blue Jay, California 92317
Phone: 800.331.8227
Internet: www.ccspublishing.com/ccs
E-mail: info@ccspublishing.com

Printed in USA                                    ISBN 978-1-934323-10-6

# Table of Contents

# *Assessment and Evaluation*

## Clinical Evaluation of the Psychiatric Patient

**I. Psychiatric History**
- **A. Identifying information.** Age, sex, marital status, race, referral source.
- **B. Chief complaint (CC).** Reason for consultation; the reason is usually a direct quote from the patient.
- **C. History of present illness (HPI)**
  1. **Current symptoms:** date of onset, duration and course of symptoms.
  2. Previous psychiatric symptoms and treatment.
  3. Recent psychosocial stressors: stressful life events that may have contributed to the patient's current presentation.
  4. Reason the patient is presenting now.
  5. This section provides evidence that supports or rules out relevant diagnoses. Therefore, documenting the absence of pertinent symptoms is also important.
  6. Historical evidence in this section should be relevant to the current presentation.
- **D. Past psychiatric history**
  1. Previous and current psychiatric diagnoses.
  2. History of psychiatric treatment, including outpatient and inpatient treatment.
  3. History of psychotropic medication use.
  4. History of suicide attempts and potential lethality.
- **E. Past medical history**
  1. Current and/or previous medical problems.
  2. Type of treatment, including prescription, over-the-counter medications, home remedies.
- **F. Family history.** Relatives with history of psychiatric disorders, suicide or suicide attempts, alcohol or substance abuse.
- **G. Social history**
  1. Source of income.
  2. Level of education, relationship history (including marriages, sexual orientation, number of children); individuals who currently live with patient.
  3. Support network.
  4. Current alcohol or illicit-drug usage.
  5. Occupational history.
- **H. Developmental history.** Family structure during childhood, relationships with parental figures and siblings; developmental milestones, peer relationships, school performance.

**II. Mental Status Exam**. The mental status exam is an assessment of the patient at the present time. Historical information should not be included in this section.
- **A. General appearance and behavior**
  1. Grooming, level of hygiene, characteristics of clothing.
  2. Unusual physical characteristics or movements.
  3. **Attitude.** Ability to interact with the interviewer.
  4. **Psychomotor activity.** Agitation or retardation.

     **5.** Degree of eye contact.
- **B. Affect**
  - **1. Definition.** External range of expression, described in terms of quality, range and appropriateness.
  - **2. Types of affect**
    - **a. Flat.** Absence of all or most affect.
    - **b. Blunted or restricted.** Moderately reduced range of affect.
    - **c. Labile.** Multiple abrupt changes in affect.
    - **d. Full or wide range of affect.** Generally appropriate.
- **C. Mood.** Internal emotional tone of the patient (ie, dysphoric, euphoric, angry, euthymic, anxious).
- **D. Thought processes**
  - **1. Use of language.** Quality and quantity of speech. The tone, associations and fluency of speech should be noted.
  - **2. Common thought disorders**
    - **a. Pressured speech.** Rapid speech, which is typical of patients with manic disorder.
    - **b. Poverty of speech.** Minimal responses, such as answering just "yes or no."
    - **c. Blocking.** Sudden cessation of speech, often in the middle of a statement.
    - **d. Flight of ideas.** Accelerated thoughts that jump from idea to idea, typical of mania.
    - **e. Loosening of associations.** Illogical shifting between unrelated topics.
    - **f. Tangentiality.** Thought that wanders from the original point.
    - **g. Circumstantiality.** Unnecessary digression, which eventually reaches the point.
    - **h. Echolalia.** Echoing of words and phrases.
    - **i. Neologisms.** Invention of new words by the patient.
    - **j. Clanging.** Speech based on sound, such as rhyming and punning rather than logical connections.
    - **k. Perseveration.** Repetition of phrases or words in the flow of speech.
    - **l. Ideas of reference.** Interpreting unrelated events as having direct reference to the patient, such as believing that the television is talking specifically to them.
- **E. Thought content**
  - **1. Definition.** Hallucinations, delusions and other perceptual disturbances.
  - **2. Common thought content disorders**
    - **a. Hallucinations.** False sensory perceptions, which may be auditory, visual, tactile, gustatory or olfactory.
    - **b. Delusions.** Fixed, false beliefs, firmly held in spite of contradictory evidence.
      - **i. Persecutory delusions.** False belief that others are trying to cause harm, or are spying with intent to cause harm.
      - **ii. Erotomanic delusions.** False belief that a person, usually of higher status, is in love with the patient.
      - **iii. Grandiose delusions.** False belief of an inflated sense of self-worth, power, knowledge, or wealth.
      - **iv. Somatic delusions.** False belief that the patient has a physical

   disorder or defect.

   c. **Illusions.** Misinterpretations of reality.
   d. **Derealization.** Feelings of unrealness involving the outer environment.
   e. **Depersonalization.** Feelings of unrealness, such as if one is "outside" of the body and observing his own activities.
   f. **Suicidal and homicidal ideation.** Suicidal and homicidal ideation requires further elaboration with comments about intent and planning (including means to carry out plan).

F. **Cognitive evaluation**
   1. **Level of consciousness.**
   2. **Orientation:** Person, place and date.
   3. **Attention and concentration:** Repeat five digits forwards and backwards or spell a five-letter word ("world") forwards and backwards.
   4. **Short-term memory:** Ability to recall three objects after five minutes.
   5. **Fund of knowledge:** Ability to name past five presidents, five large cities, or historical dates.
   6. **Calculations.** Subtraction of serial 7s, simple math problems.
   7. **Abstraction.** Proverb interpretation and similarities.

G. **Insight.** Ability of the patient to display an understanding of his current problems, and the ability to understand the implication of these problems.

H. **Judgment.** Ability to make sound decisions regarding everyday activities. Judgement is best evaluated by assessing a patient's history of decision making, rather than by asking hypothetical questions.

III. **DSM-IV Multiaxial Assessment Diagnosis**

   **Axis I:**   Clinical disorders.
   Other conditions that may be a focus of clinical attention.

   **Axis II:**  Personality disorders.
   Mental retardation.

   **Axis III:** General medical conditions.

   **Axis IV:** Psychosocial and environmental problems.

   **Axis V:**  Global assessment of functioning.

IV. **Treatment plan.** This section should discuss pharmacologic treatment and other psychiatric therapy, including hospitalization.

V. **General medical screening of the psychiatric patient.** A thorough physical and neurological examination, including basic screening laboratory studies to rule out physical conditions, should be completed.

A. **Laboratory evaluation of the psychiatric patient**
   1. CBC with differential.
   2. Blood chemistry (SMAC).
   3. Thyroid function panel.
   4. Screening test for syphilis (RPR or MHA-TP).
   5. Urinalysis with drug screen.
   6. Urine pregnancy check for females of childbearing potential.
   7. Blood alcohol level.
   8. Serum levels of medications.
   9. Hepatitis C testing in at-risk patients.
   10. HIV test in high-risk patients.

B. A more extensive work-up and laboratory studies may be indicated based on clinical findings.

# Admitting Orders

**Admit to:** (Name of unit).
**Diagnosis:** DSM-IV diagnosis justifying the admit.
**Legal Status:** Voluntary or involuntary status- if involuntary, state specific status.
**Condition:** Stable.
**Allergies:** No known allergies.
**Vitals:** Standard orders are q shift x 3, then q day if stable; if there are medical concerns, vitals should be ordered more frequently.
**Activity:** Restrict to the unit or allow patient to leave unit.
**Precautions:** Assault or suicide precautions, elopement precautions.
**Diet:** Regular diet, ADA diet, soft mechanical.
**Labs:** Chem 20, CBC with diff, UA with toxicology screen, urine pregnancy test, RPR, thyroid function, serum levels of medications.
**Medications:** As indicated by the patient's diagnosis or target symptoms. Include as-needed medications, such as Tylenol, milk of magnesia, antacids.

# Schizophrenia Admitting Orders

**Admit to:** Acute Psychiatric Unit.
**Diagnosis:** Schizophrenia, Continuous Paranoid Type, Acute Exacerbation.
**Legal Status:** Involuntary by conservator.
**Condition:** Actively Psychotic.
**Allergies:** No known allergies.
**Vitals:** q shift x 3, then q day if stable.
**Activity:** Restrict to unit.
**Precautions:** Assault precautions.
**Diet:** Regular.
**Labs:** Chem 20, CBC with diff, UA with toxicology screen, urine pregnancy test, RPR, thyroid function.
**Medications:**
 Risperidone (Risperdal) 2 mg po bid x 2 days, then 4 mg po qhs.
 Lorazepam (Ativan) 2 mg po q 4 hours prn agitation (not to exceed 8 mg/24 hours.
 Zolpidem (Ambien) 10 mg po qhs prn insomnia.
 Tylenol 650 mg po q 4 hours prn pain or fever.
 Milk of magnesia 30 cc po q 12 hours prn constipation.
 Mylanta 30 cc po q 4 hours prn dyspepsia.

# Bipolar I Disorder Admitting Orders

**Admit to:** Acute Psychiatric Unit.
**Diagnosis:** Bipolar I Disorder, Manic with psychotic features.
**Legal Status:** Involuntary (legal hold, 5150 in California).
**Condition:** Actively Psychotic.
**Allergies:** No known allergies.
**Vitals:** q shift x 3, then q day if stable.
**Activity:** Restrict to unit.

**Precautions:** Elopement precautions.
**Diet:** Regular.
**Labs**: Chem 20, CBC with diff, UA with toxicology screen, urine pregnancy test, RPR, thyroid function, valproate level.
**Medications:**
  Aripiprazole (Abilify) 10 mg po qd.
  Lorazepam (Ativan) 2 mg po q 4 hours prn agitation (not to exceed 8 mg/24 hours.
  Depakote 500 mg po tid.
  Zaleplon (Sonata) 10 mg po qhs prn insomnia.
  Tylenol 650 mg po q 4 hours prn pain or fever.
  Milk of magnesia 30 cc po q 12 hours prn constipation.
  Mylanta 30 cc po q 4 hours prn dyspepsia.

## Major Depression Admitting Orders

**Admit to:** Acute Psychiatric Unit.
**Diagnosis:** Major Depression, severe, without psychotic features.
**Legal Status:** Voluntary.
**Condition:** Stable.
**Allergies:** No known allergies.
**Vitals:** q shift x 3, then q day if stable.
**Activity:** Restrict to unit.
**Precautions:** Suicide precautions.
**Diet:** Regular.
**Labs:** Chem 20, CBC with diff, UA with toxicology screen, urine pregnancy test, RPR, thyroid function.
**Medications:**
  Sertraline (Zoloft) 50 mg po qAM.
  Lorazepam (Ativan) 2 mg po q 4 hours prn agitation (not to exceed 8 mg/24 hours.
  Trazodone (Desyrel) 50 mg po qhs prn insomnia.
  Tylenol 650 mg po q 4 hours prn pain or fever.
  Milk of magnesia 30 cc po q 12 hours prn constipation.
  Mylanta 30 cc po q 4 hours prn dyspepsia.

## Alcohol Dependence Admitting Orders

**Admit to:** Alcohol Treatment Unit.
**Diagnosis:** Alcohol Dependence.
**Legal Status:** Voluntary.
**Condition:** Guarded.
**Allergies:** No known allergies.
**Vitals:** q shift x 3 days, then q day if stable.
**Activity:** Restrict to unit.
**Precautions:** Seizure and withdrawal precautions.
**Diet:** Regular with one can of Ensure with each meal.
**Labs:** Chem 20, CBC with diff, UA with toxicology screen, urine pregnancy test, RPR, thyroid function.

**Medications:**
Folate 1 mg po qd.
Thiamine 100 mg IM qd x 3 days, then 100 mg po qd.
Multivitamin 1 po qd.
Lorazepam (Ativan) 2 mg po tid x 2 days, then 2 mg bid x 2 days, then 1 mg po bid x 2 days, then discontinue.
Lorazepam (Ativan) 2 mg po q 4 hours prn alcohol withdrawal symptoms (pulse >100, systolic BP >160, diastolic BP >100 [not to exceed 14 mg/24 hour]).
Zolpidem (Ambien) 10 mg po qhs prn insomnia.
Tylenol 650 mg po q 4 hours prn pain or fever.
Milk of magnesia 30 cc po q 12 hours prn constipation.
Mylanta 30 cc po q 4 hours prn dyspepsia.

# Opiate Dependence Admitting Orders

**Admit to:** Acute Psychiatric Unit.
**Diagnosis:** Heroin dependance.
**Legal Status:** Voluntary.
**Condition:** Stable.
**Allergies:** No known allergies.
**Vitals:** q shift x 3 days, then q day if stable.
**Activity:** Restrict to unit.
**Precautions:** Opiate withdrawal.
**Diet:** Regular.
**Labs:** Chem 20, CBC with diff, UA with toxicology screen, urine pregnancy test, RPR, thyroid function, hepatitis panel, HIV.
**Medications:**
Clonidine (Catapres) 0.1 mg po qid, hold for systolic BP <90 or diastolic BP <60). Give 0.1 mg po q 4 hours prn signs and symptoms of opiate withdrawal.
Dicyclomine (Bentyl) 20 mg po q 6 hours prn cramping.
Ibuprofen (Advil) 600 mg po q 6 hours prn pain/headache.
Methocarbamol (Robaxin) 500 mg po q 6 hours prn muscle pain.
Lorazepam (Ativan) 2 mg po q 4 hours prn agitation (not to exceed 8 mg/24 hours.
Zolpidem (Ambien) 10 mg po qhs prn insomnia.
Milk of magnesia 30 cc po q 12 hours prn constipation.
Mylanta 30 cc po q 4 hours prn dyspepsia.

# Schizoaffective Disorder Admitting Orders

**Admit to:** Acute Psychiatric Unit.
**Diagnosis:** Schizoaffective disorder, bipolar type, depressed.
**Legal Status:** Voluntary.
**Condition:** Stable.
**Allergies:** No known allergies.
**Vitals:** q shift x 3, then q day if stable.
**Activity:** Restrict to unit.
**Precautions:** Suicide precautions.

**Diet:** Regular.
**Labs:** Chem 20, CBC with diff, UA with toxicology screen, urine pregnancy test, RPR, thyroid function, lithium level.
**Medications:**
  Quetiapine (Seroquel) 100 mg po bid x 2 days, then 200 mg po bid.
  Lithium 600 mg po bid.
  Citalopram (Celexa) 20 mg po q am.
  Lorazepam (Ativan) 2 mg po q 4 hours prn agitation (not to exceed 8 mg/24 hours).
  Zolpidem (Ambien) 10 mg po qhs prn insomnia.
  Tylenol 650 mg po q 4 hours prn pain or fever.
  Milk of magnesia 30 cc po q 12 hours prn constipation.
  Mylanta 30 cc po q 4 hours prn dyspepsia.

# Restraint Orders

1. **Type of Restraint:** Seclusion, 4-point leather restraint, or soft restraints.
2. **Indication:**
   Confused, threat to self.
   Agitated, threat to self.
   Combative, threat to self/others.
   Attempting to pull out tube, line, or dressing.
   Attempting to get out of bed, fall risk.
3. **Time**
   Begin at _____ o'clock.
   Not to exceed (specify number of hours).
4. Monitor patient as directed by hospital policy.
5. Staff may decrease or release restraints at their discretion.

# Restraint Notes

The restraint note should document that less restrictive measures were attempted and failed or were considered, but not appropriate for the urgent clinical situation.

---

**Restraint Note**

**Date/time/writer:**
The patient became agitated and, without provocation, threw a chair and threatened several patients verbally. He was unmanageable; therefore, immediate 4-point restraints were required. Other less-restrictive measures, such as locked seclusion, were considered but deemed inappropriate given his severe agitation and assaultive behavior. He will be observed per protocol and may be released at staff's discretion. He will be given haloperidol (Haldol) 10 mg IM and lorazepam (Ativan) 2 mg IM because he has refused oral medication.

# Psychiatric Progress Notes

Daily progress notes should summarize the patient's current clinical condition and should review developments in the patient's hospital course. The note should address problems that remain active, plans to treat those problems, and arrangements for discharge. Progress notes should address every element of the problem list.

---

## Psychiatric Progress Note

**Date/time/writer:**
**Subjective:** A direct quote from the patient should be written in the chart. Information reported by the patient may include complaints, symptoms, side effects, life events, and feelings.
**Objective:**
Discuss pertinent clinical events and observations of the nursing staff.
**Affect:** Flat, blunted, labile, full.
**Mood:** Dysphoric, euphoric, angry, euthymic, anxious.
**Thought Processes:** Quality and quantity of speech. Tone, associations and fluency of speech, and speech abnormalities.
**Thought Content:** Hallucinations, paranoid ideation, suicidal ideation.
**Cognitive:** Orientation, attention, concentration.
**Insight:** Ability of the patient understand his current problems
**Judgment:** Decision-making ability.
**Labs:** New test results.
**Current medications:** List medications and dosages.
**Assessment:** This section should be organized by problem. A separate assessment should be written for each problem (eg, stable or actively psychotic). Documentation of dangerousness to self or others should be addressed. The assessment should include reasons that support the patient's continuing need for hospitalization. Documentation may include suicidality, homicidality, informed consent issues, monitoring of medication side effects (eg, serum drug levels, WBCs, abnormal involuntary movements).
**Plan:** Changes to current treatment, future considerations, and issues that require continued monitoring should be discussed.

### Inpatient Progress Note

**Date/time/Psychiatry R2**
**S:** "The FBI is trying to kill me." The patient reports that she was unable to sleep last night because the FBI harassed her by talking to her. She became frightened during our interview and refused to talk after 5 minutes.
**O:** The patient slept for only 2 hours last night and refused to take medications, which were offered to her. Patient is also reluctant to eat or drink fearing that the food is poisoned. On exam, the patient displayed poor eye contact, and psychomotor agitation.
  **Affect:** Flat.
  **Mood:** Dysphoric.
  **Thought Processes:** Speech is limited to a few paranoid statements about the FBI. Otherwise the patient remains electively mute.
  **Thought Content:** Auditory hallucinations and paranoid ideation. The patient denies visual hallucination, suicidal ideation. The patient denies homicidal ideation, but states that she would harm anyone from the FBI who tried to hurt her.
  **Cognitive:** The patient would not answer orientation questions due to paranoid ideation.
  **Insight:** Poor.
  **Judgment:** Impaired.
**A:** 1. Schizophrenia, chronic, paranoid type with acute exacerbation. The patient is actively psychotic and paranoid, with extensive impact on functioning.
**P:** 1. The patient remains actively paranoid and intermittently compliant with recommended medication. Continue to encourage patient to take medication, Risperdal 2 mg PO BID.
   2. Continue to monitor sleep, food and fluid intake. Draw electrolyte panel in the AM to monitor hydration status.
   3. **Legal Status:** The patient is currently hospitalized on an involuntary basis. The patient meets criteria for involuntary hospitalization due to an inability to provide food, clothing and shelter for herself.

## Discharge Note

The discharge note should be written in the patient's chart prior to discharge.

### Discharge Note

**Date/time:**
**Diagnoses:**
**Treatment:** Briefly describe therapy provided during hospitalization, including psychiatric drug therapy, and medical/surgical consultations and treatment.
**Studies Performed:** Electrocardiograms, CT scan, psychological testing.
**Discharge Medications:**
**Follow-up Arrangements:**

# Discharge Summary

The discharge summary reviews how a patient presented to the hospital, salient psychosocial information, and the course of treatment, diagnostic tests and response to interventions are also discussed.

**Patient's Name and Medical Record Number:**
**Date of Admission:**
**Date of Discharge:**
**DSM-IV Multiaxial Discharge Diagnosis**
- **Axis I:** Clinical disorders.
  Other conditions that may be a focus of clinical attention.
- **Axis II:** Personality disorders.
- **Axis III:** Medical conditions.
- **Axis IV:** Psychosocial and environmental problems.
- **Axis V:** Global assessment of functioning.

**Attending or Ward Team Responsible for Patient:**
**Surgical Procedures, Diagnostic Tests, Invasive Procedures:**
**History of Present Illness:** Include salient features surrounding reason for admission, past psychiatric history, social history, mental status exam and physical examination.
**Diagnostic Data:** Results of laboratory testing, psychological testing, and brain imaging.
**Hospital Course:** Describe the course of the patient's illness while in the hospital, including evaluation, consultations, medications, outcome of treatment, and unresolved issues at discharge. All items on the problem list should be addressed.
**Discharged Condition:** Describe improvement or deterioration in the patient's condition, and describe the present status of the patient.
**Disposition:** Describe the situation to which the patient will be discharged (home, nursing home), and indicate who will take care of patient.
**Legal Status at Discharge**: Voluntary, involuntary, conservatorship.
**Discharge Medications:** List medications, dosages, quantities dispensed, and instructions.
**Discharge Instructions and Follow-up Care:** Date of return for follow-up care at clinic; diet, exercise.
**Copies:** Send copies to attending, clinic, consultants.

> **Outpatient Progress Note**
>
> **Subjective**: The patient reports improved mood, sleep, and appetite, but energy remains low. The patient denies any side effects of medications other than mild nausea that has been diminishing over the past few days. The patient's spouse reports increased interest in usual activities.
>
> **Objective**: The patient is casually dressed with good grooming. Speech is more spontaneous, but output is decreased. Mood remains depressed but improved from the previous visit. Affect is brighter but still constricted. Thinking is logical and goal directed. The patient denies any recent suicidal or homicidal ideation. No psychotic symptoms are noted. Cognition is grossly intact. Insight is improving, and judgment remains good.
>
> **Assessment**: Major depression is improving with nefazodone and supportive psychotherapy, but the patient still has symptoms after 4 weeks of treatment at 200 mg bid.
>
> **Plan:** Increase nefazodone from 200 mg bid to 200 mg q AM and 400 mg qhs. Continue weekly supportive therapy. Refer to senior center for increased social interaction.

# Psychological Testing

Psychological testing often provides additional information that complements the psychiatric history and mental status exam.

I.   **Psychological tests characterize psychological symptoms, as well as describe personality and motivations.**
    A.  **Rorschach Test.** Ink blots serve as stimuli for free associations; particularly helpful in psychodynamic formulation and assessment of defense mechanisms and ego boundaries.
    B.  **Thematic Apperception Test (TAT).** The patient is asked to consider pictures of people in a variety of situations, and is asked to make up a story for each card. This test provides information about needs, conflicts, defenses, fantasies, and interpersonal relationships.
    C.  **Sentence Completion Test (SCT).** Patients are asked to finish incomplete sentences, thereby revealing conscious associations. Provides insight into defenses, fears and preoccupations of the patient.
    D.  **Minnesota Multiphasic Personality Inventory (MMPI).** A battery of questions assessing personality characteristics. Results are given in 10 scales.
    E.  **Draw-a-Person Test (DAP).** The patient is asked to draw a picture of a person, and then to draw a picture of a person of the opposite sex of the first drawing. The drawings represent how the patient relates to his environment, and the test may also be used as a screening exam for brain damage.
II.  **Neuropsychological tests assess cognitive abilities and can assist in characterizing impaired brain function.**
    A.  **Bender Gestalt Test.** A test of visual-motor and spatial abilities, useful for children and adults.
    B.  **Halstead-Reitan Battery and Luria-Nebraska Inventory**
        1.  Standardized evaluation of brain functioning.

2. Assess expressive and receptive language, memory, intellectual reasoning and judgment, visual-motor function, sensory-perceptual function and motor function.

C. **Wechsler Adult Intelligence Scale (WAIS).** Intelligence test that measures verbal IQ, performance IQ, and full-scale IQ.

D. **Wisconsin Card Sort.** A test of frontal lobe function.

*References*
References, see page 120.

# Psychotic Disorders

## Schizophrenia

Schizophrenia is a disorder characterized by apathy, absence of initiative (avolition), and affective blunting. These patients have alterations in thoughts, perceptions, mood, and behavior. Many schizophrenics display delusions, hallucinations and misinterpretations of reality.

### I. DSM-IV Diagnostic Criteria for Schizophrenia
  **A.** Two or more of the following symptoms present for one month:
  1. Delusions.
  2. Hallucinations.
  3. Disorganized speech.
  4. Grossly disorganized or catatonic behavior.
  5. Negative symptoms (ie, affective flattening, alogia, avolition).

  **B.** Decline in social and/or occupational functioning since the onset of illness.

  **C.** Continuous signs of illness for at least six months with at least one month of active symptoms.

  **D.** Schizoaffective disorder and mood disorder with psychotic features have been excluded.

  **E.** The disturbance is not due to substance abuse or a medical condition.

  **F.** If history of autistic disorder or pervasive developmental disorder is present, schizophrenia may be diagnosed only if prominent delusions or hallucinations have been present for one month.

### II. Clinical Features of Schizophrenia
  **A.** A prior history of schizotypal or schizoid personality traits or disorder is often present.

  **B.** Symptoms of schizophrenia have been traditionally categorized as either positive or negative. Depression and neurocognitive dysfunction are gaining acceptance as terms to describe two other core symptoms of schizophrenia.

  1. **Positive symptoms**
     a. Hallucinations are most commonly auditory or visual, but hallucinations can occur in any sensory modality.
     b. Delusions.
     c. Disorganized behavior.
     d. Thought disorder is characterized by loose associations, tangentiality, incoherent thoughts, neologisms, thought blocking, thought insertion, thought broadcasting, and ideas of reference.

  2. **Negative symptoms**
     a. Poverty of speech (alogia) or poverty of thought content.
     b. Anhedonia.
     c. Flat affect.
     d. Loss of motivation (avolition).
     e. Attentional deficits.
     f. Loss of social interest.

  3. **Depression** is common and often severe in schizophrenia and can compromise functional status and response to treatment. Atypical antipsychotics often improve depressive signs and symptoms, but

      antidepressants may be required.

    **4. Cognitive impairment.** Cognitive dysfunction (including attention, executive function, and particular types of memory) contribute to disability and can be an obstacle in long-term treatment. Atypical antipsychotics may improve cognitive impairment.

  **C.** The presence of tactile, olfactory or gustatory hallucinations may indicate an organic etiology such as complex partial seizures.

  **D.** Sensorium is intact.

  **E.** Insight and judgment are frequently impaired.

  **F.** No sign or symptom is pathognomonic of schizophrenia.

## III. Epidemiology of Schizophrenia

  **A.** The lifetime prevalence of schizophrenia is one percent.

  **B.** Onset of psychosis usually occurs in the late teens or early twenties.

  **C.** Males and females are equally affected, but the mean age of onset is approximately six years later in females. Females frequently have a milder course of illness.

  **D.** The suicide rate is 10-13%, similar to the rate that occurs in depressive illnesses. More than 75% of patients are smokers, and the incidence of substance abuse is increased (especially alcohol, cocaine, methamphetamine and marijuana).

  **E.** Most patients follow a chronic downward course, but some have a gradual improvement with a decrease in positive symptoms and increased functioning. Very few patients have a complete recovery.

  **F.** The lifespan for patients with schizophrenia is approximately 10 years shorter compared to the general population. This is thought to be related to lifestyle (poor nutrition, lack of exercise, smoking substance abuse), decreased access to medical care and higher suicide rate.

## IV. Classification of Schizophrenia

  **A. Paranoid type Schizophrenia**

    **1.** Characterized by a preoccupation with one or more delusions or frequent auditory hallucinations.

    **2.** Paranoid type schizophrenia is characterized by the absence of prominent disorganization of speech, disorganized or catatonic behavior, or flat or inappropriate affect.

  **B. Disorganized type Schizophrenia** is characterized by prominent disorganized speech, disorganized behavior, and flat or inappropriate affect.

  **C. Catatonic type Schizophrenia** is characterized by at least two of the following:

    **1.** Motoric immobility.

    **2.** Excessive motor activity.

    **3.** Extreme negativism or mutism.

    **4.** Peculiar voluntary movements such as bizarre posturing.

    **5.** Echolalia or echopraxia.

  **D. Undifferentiated type Schizophrenia** meets criteria for schizophrenia, but it cannot be characterized as paranoid, disorganized, or catatonic type.

  **E. Residual type Schizophrenia** is characterized by the absence of prominent delusions, disorganized speech and grossly disorganized or catatonic behavior and continued negative symptoms or two or more attenuated positive symptoms.

## V. Differential Diagnosis of Schizophrenia

A. **Psychotic disorder due to a general medical condition, delirium, or dementia.** Included would be CNS infections, thyrotoxicosis, lupus, myxedema, multiple strokes, HIV, hepatic encephalopathy, and others.

B. **Substance-induced psychotic disorder.** Amphetamines and cocaine frequently cause hallucinations, paranoia, or delusions. Phencyclidine (PCP) may lead to both positive and negative symptoms.

C. **Schizoaffective disorder.** Mood symptoms are present for a significant portion of the illness. In schizophrenia, the duration of mood symptoms is brief compared to the entire duration of the illness.

D. **Mood disorder with psychotic features**
   1. Psychotic symptoms occur only during major mood disturbance (mania or major depression).
   2. Disturbances of mood are frequent in all phases of schizophrenia.

E. **Delusional disorder.** Non-bizarre delusions are present in the absence of other psychotic symptoms.

F. **Schizotypal, paranoid, schizoid or borderline personality disorders**
   1. Psychotic symptoms are generally mild and brief in duration.
   2. Patterns of behavior are life-long, with no identifiable time of onset.

G. **Brief psychotic disorder.** Duration of symptoms is between one day to one month.

H. **Schizophreniform disorder.** The criteria for schizophrenia are met, but the duration of illness is less than six months.

## VI. Treatment of Schizophrenia

A. **Pharmacotherapy.** Antipsychotic medications reduce core symptoms and are the cornerstone of treatment of schizophrenia.

B. Psychosocial treatments in conjunction with medications are often indicated. Day treatment programs, with emphasis on social skills training, can improve functioning and decrease relapse.

C. A complete discussion of the treatment of Schizophrenia can be found on page 96.

D. Family therapy and individual supportive psychotherapy are also useful in relapse prevention.

E. Electroconvulsive therapy is rarely used in the treatment of schizophrenia, but may be useful when catatonia or prominent affective symptoms are present.

F. **Indications for hospitalization**
   1. Psychotic symptoms prevent the patient from caring for his basic needs.
   2. Suicidal ideation, secondary to psychosis, often requires hospitalization.
   3. Patients who are a danger to themselves or others require hospitalization.
   4. Patients with command hallucinations to harm self or others should be evaluated for hospitalization, especially with a history of acting on hallucinations.

# Schizoaffective Disorder

## I. DSM-IV Diagnostic Criteria
   **A.** Schizoaffective disorder is an illness, which meets the criteria for schizophrenia and concurrently meets the criteria for a major depressive episode, manic episode, or mixed episode.
   **B.** The illness must also be associated with delusions or hallucinations for two weeks, without significant mood symptoms.
   **C.** Mood symptoms must be present for a significant portion of the illness.
   **D.** A general medical condition or substance use is not the cause of symptoms.

## II. Clinical Features of Schizoaffective Disorder
   **A.** Symptoms of schizophrenia are present, but the symptoms are also associated with recurrent or chronic mood disturbances.
   **B.** Psychotic symptoms and mood symptoms may occur independently or together.
   **C.** If manic or mixed symptoms occur, they must be present for one week, and major depressive symptoms must be present for two weeks.

## III. Epidemiology of Schizoaffective Disorder
   **A.** The lifetime prevalence is under one percent.
   **B.** First-degree biological relatives of schizoaffective disorder patients have an increased risk of schizophrenia as well as mood disorders.

## IV. Classification of Schizoaffective Disorder
   **A. Bipolar Type.** Diagnosed when a manic or mixed episode occurs. Major depression may also occur.
   **B. Depressive type.** Diagnosed if only major depressive episodes occur.

## V. Differential Diagnosis of Schizoaffective Disorder
   **A. Schizophrenia.** In schizophrenia, mood symptoms are relatively brief in relation to psychotic symptoms. Mood symptoms usually do not meet the full criteria for major depressive or manic episodes.
   **B. Mood disorder with psychotic features.** In mood disorder with psychotic features, the psychotic features occur only in the presence of a major mood disturbance.
   **C. Delusional Disorder.** Depressive symptoms can occur in delusional disorders, but psychotic symptoms of a delusional disorder are non-bizarre compared to schizoaffective disorder.
   **D. Substance-Induced Psychotic Disorder.** Psychotic and mood symptoms of schizoaffective disorder can also be mimicked by street drugs, medications, or toxins.
   **E. Psychotic disorder due to a general medical condition, delirium, or dementia** should be ruled out by medical history, physical exam, and labs.

## VI. Treatment of Schizoaffective Disorder
   **A.** Psychotic symptoms are treated with antipsychotic agents (see Antipsychotic Therapy, page 96).
   **B.** The depressed phase of schizoaffective disorder is treated with antidepressant medications (see Antidepressant Therapy, page 105).
   **C.** For bipolar type, mood stabilizers (eg, lithium, valproate or carbamazepine) are used alone or in combination with antipsychotics (see Mood Stabilizers, page 110).
   **D.** Electroconvulsive therapy may be necessary for severe depression or mania.

  **E.** Hospitalization and supportive psychotherapy may be required.

# Schizophreniform Disorder

Patients with schizophreniform disorder meet full criteria for schizophrenia, but the duration of illness is between one and six months.

**I. DSM-IV Diagnostic Criteria for Schizophreniform Disorder**
  **A. The following criteria for schizophrenia must be met:**
    1. Two or more symptoms for one month. Symptoms may include delusions, hallucinations, disorganized speech, grossly disorganized or catatonic behavior, or negative symptoms.
    2. Schizoaffective disorder and mood disorder with psychotic features must be excluded.
    3. Substance-induced symptoms or symptoms from a general medical condition have been ruled out.
    4. Symptomatology must last for at least one month, but less than six months.
**II. Clinical Features of Schizophreniform Disorder**
  **A.** Symptomatology, including positive and negative psychotic features, is the same as schizophrenia.
  **B.** Social and occupational functioning may or may not be impaired.
**III. Epidemiology of Schizophreniform Disorder**
  **A.** Lifetime prevalence of schizophreniform disorder is approximately 0.2%.
  **B.** Prevalence is the same in males and females.
  **C.** Depressive symptoms commonly coexist and are associated with an increased suicide risk.
**IV. Classification of Schizophreniform Disorder**
  **A. Schizophreniform disorder with good prognostic features**
    1. Onset of psychosis occurs within four weeks of behavioral change.
    2. Confusion often present at peak of psychosis.
    3. Good premorbid social and occupational functioning.
    4. Lack of blunted or flat affect.
  **B.** Schizophreniform disorder without good prognostic features is characterized by the absence of above features.
**V. Differential Diagnosis of Schizophreniform Disorder**
  **A.** The differential diagnosis for schizophreniform disorder is the same as for schizophrenia and includes psychotic disorder due to a general medical condition, delirium, or dementia.
  **B.** Substance abuse, medication or toxic substances may cause symptoms that are similar to schizophreniform disorder.
  **C.** Concomitant use of drugs that can cause or exacerbate psychosis, such as amphetamines, may complicate the diagnostic process.
**VI. Treatment of Schizophreniform Disorder**
  **A.** Antipsychotic medication in conjunction with supportive psychotherapy is the primary treatment (see Antipsychotic Therapy, page 96).
  **B.** Hospitalization may be required if the patient is unable to care for himself or if suicidal or homicidal ideation is present.
  **C.** Depressive symptoms may require antidepressants or mood stabilizers.
  **D.** Early and aggressive treatment is associated with a better prognosis.

# Brief Psychotic Disorder

Brief psychotic disorder is characterized by hallucinations, delusions, disorganized speech or behavior. Symptom onset is often rapid, with marked functional impairment. The duration of symptoms is between one day and one month. In contrast, diagnosis of schizophrenia requires a six-month duration of symptoms.

## I. DSM-IV Diagnostic Criteria for Brief Psychotic Disorder
   A. **At least one of the following:**
      1. Delusions.
      2. Hallucinations.
      3. Disorganized speech.
      4. Grossly disorganized or catatonic behavior.
   B. Duration of symptoms is between one day and one month, after which the patient returns to the previous level of functioning.
   C. The disturbance is not caused by a mood disorder with psychotic features, substance abuse, schizoaffective disorder, schizophrenia, or other medical condition.

## II. Clinical Features of Brief Psychotic Disorder
   A. Emotional turmoil and confusion are often present.
   B. Mood and affect may be labile.
   C. Onset is usually sudden and may abate as rapidly as it began.
   D. Attentional deficits are common.
   E. Psychotic symptoms are usually of brief duration (several days).

## III. Epidemiology of Brief Psychotic Disorder
   A. The disorder is rare, and younger individuals have a higher rate of illness, with the average age of onset in the late twenties to early thirties.
   B. The risk of suicide is increased in patients with this disorder, especially in young patients.
   C. Patients with personality disorders have a higher risk for brief psychotic disorder.

## IV. Classification of Brief Psychotic Disorder
   A. **Brief Psychotic Disorder with Marked Stressors** is present if symptoms occur in relation to severe stressors (ie, death of a loved one).
   B. **Brief Psychotic Disorder without Marked Stressors** is present if symptoms occur without identifiable stressors.
   C. **Brief Psychotic Disorder with Postpartum Onset** occurs within four weeks of giving birth.

## V. Differential Diagnosis of Brief Psychotic Disorder
   A. **Substance-Induced Psychotic Disorder**
      1. Amphetamine, cocaine and PCP may produce symptoms indistinguishable from brief psychotic disorder. Alcohol or sedative hypnotic withdrawal may also mimic these symptoms.
      2. Substance abuse should be excluded by history and with a urine toxicology screen.
   B. **Psychotic Disorder Caused a General Medical Condition**
      1. Rule out with history, physical exam and labs. A CBC can be used to rule out delirium and psychosis caused by infection. This is especially important in elderly patients where the incidence of brief reactive psychosis is low compared to younger patients.
      2. Routine chemistry labs can be used to rule out electrolyte imbalances

or hepatic encephalopathy; RPR to rule out neurosyphilis; HIV to rule out psychosis due to encephalitis in at-risk patients.

  3. Consider an MRI or head CT scan to rule out a mass or neoplasm.
  4. An EEG should be considered to rule out seizure disorders (such as temporal lobe epilepsy), especially when there is a history of amnestic periods or impaired consciousness.

C. **Schizophreniform Disorder or Schizophrenia.** Schizophreniform disorder must last for over a month, and schizophrenia must have a six-month duration.

D. **Mood Disorder with Psychotic Features.** Brief psychotic disorder cannot be diagnosed if the full criteria for major depressive, manic or mixed episode is present

## VI. Treatment of Brief Psychotic Disorder

A. Brief hospitalization may be necessary, especially if suicidal or homicidal ideation is present. Patients can also be very confused and impulsive.

B. A brief course of a neuroleptic, such as risperidone (Risperdal) 2-4 mg per day, is usually indicated. Adjunctive benzodiazepines can speed the resolution of symptoms. Short-acting benzodiazepines, such as lorazepam 1-2 mg every 4 to 6 hours, can be used as needed for associated agitation and anxiety.

C. Supportive psychotherapy is indicated if precipitating stressors are present. Supportive psychotherapy is initiated after psychosis has resolved.

# Delusional Disorder

Delusional disorder is characterized by the presence of irrational, untrue beliefs.

## I. DSM-IV Diagnostic Criteria for Delusional Disorder

A. Non-bizarre delusions have lasted for at least one month.

B. This disorder is characterized by the absence of hallucinations, disorganized speech, grossly disorganized or catatonic behavior, or negative symptoms of schizophrenia (tactile or olfactory hallucinations may be present if related to the delusional theme).

C. Behavior and functioning are not significantly bizarre or impaired.

D. If mood episodes have occurred, the total duration of mood pathology is brief compared to the duration of the delusions.

## II. Clinical Features of Delusional Disorder

A. The presence of a non-bizarre delusion is the cardinal feature of this disorder. The delusion must be plausible, such as believing that someone is trying to harm them.

B. Patient's thought processes and thought content are normal except when discussing the specific delusion.

C. Hallucinations are not prominent unless delusional disorder is of the somatic type. Cognition and sensorium are intact.

D. There is generally no disturbance of thought processes, such as loosening of associations or tangentiality.

E. The insight of patients into their illness is generally poor, and this disorder may cause significant impairment in social and occupational functioning.

## III. Epidemiology of Delusional Disorder

A. Delusional disorder is uncommon, with a prevalence of 0.03%.

**B.** Mean age of onset is generally between 35-45; however, age of onset is highly variable. The incidence in males and females appears equal.

## IV. Classification of Delusional Disorder

**A. Persecutory type.** Involves delusions that the individual is being harassed.

**B. Somatic type.** Involves delusions of a physical deficit or medical condition.

**C. Erotomanic type.** Involves delusions that another person is in love with the patient.

**D. Grandiose type.** Involves delusions of exaggerated power, wealth, knowledge, identity or relationship to a famous person or religious figure.

**E. Jealous type.** Involves delusions that an individual's partner is unfaithful.

**F. Mixed type.** Involves delusions of at least two of the above without a predominate theme.

## V. Differential Diagnosis of Delusional Disorder

**A. Schizophrenia/Schizophreniform Disorder.** Delusional disorder is distinguished from these disorders by a lack of other positive or negative symptoms of psychosis.

**B. Substance-Induced Psychotic Disorder**
1. Symptoms may be identical to delusional disorder if the patient has ingested amphetamines or cocaine.
2. Substance abuse should be excluded by history and toxicology.

**C. Psychotic Disorder Due to a General Medical Condition**
1. Simple delusions of a persecutory or somatic nature are often present in delirium or dementia.
2. Cognitive exam, history and physical examination can usually distinguish these conditions.

**D. Mood Disorders With Psychotic Features.** Although mood symptoms and delusions may be present in both disorders, patients with delusional disorder do not meet full criteria for a mood episode, and the duration of mood symptoms is brief compared to delusional symptoms.

## VI. Treatment of Delusional Disorder

**A.** Delusional disorders are often refractory to antipsychotic medication.

**B.** Psychotherapy, including family or couples therapy, may offer some benefit.

### References
References, see page 120.

# *Mood Disorders*

I. **Categorization of Mood Disorders**
   A. **Mood episodes** are comprised of periods when the patient exhibits symptoms of a predominant mood state. Mood episodes are not diagnostic entities. The mood disorders are clinical diagnoses defined by the presence of characteristic mood episodes.
   B. **Mood episodes are classified as follows:**
      1. **Types of Mood Episodes**
         a. Major Depressive Episode.
         b. Manic Episode.
         c. Mixed Episode.
         d. Hypomanic Episode.
   C. **Mood disorders are classified as follows:**
      1. **Types of Mood Disorders**
         a. Depressive Disorders.
         b. Bipolar Disorders.
         c. Other Mood Disorders.

## Major Depressive Episodes

Major depressive episodes are characterized by persistent sadness, often associated with somatic symptoms, such as weight loss, difficulty sleeping and decreased energy.

I. **DSM-IV Diagnostic Criteria**
   A. At least five of the following symptoms for at least two weeks duration.
   B. Must be a change from previous functioning.
   C. At least one symptom is depressed mood or loss of interest or pleasure.
      1. Pervasive depressed mood.
      2. Pervasive anhedonia.
      3. Significant change in weight.
      4. Sleep disturbance.
      5. Psychomotor agitation or retardation.
      6. Pervasive fatigue or loss of energy.
      7. Excessive guilt or feelings of worthlessness.
      8. Difficulty concentrating.
      9. Recurrent thoughts of death or thoughts of suicide.
   D. Symptoms must cause significant social or occupational dysfunction or significant subjective distress.
   E. Cannot be caused by a medical condition, medication or drugs.
   F. Symptoms cannot be caused by bereavement.
II. **Clinical Features of Depressive Episodes**
   A. Occasionally no subjective depressed mood is present; only anxiety and irritability are displayed.
   B. Feelings of hopelessness and helplessness are common.
   C. Decreased libido is common.
   D. Early morning awakening with difficulty or inability to fall back asleep is typical.

E. Psychomotor agitation can be severe.
F. Patients may appear demented because of poor attention, poor concentration, and indecisiveness.
G. Guilt may become excessive and may appear delusional.
H. Obsessive rumination about the past or specific problems is common.
I. Preoccupation with physical health may occur.
J. Frank delusions and hallucinations may occur, and they are frequently nihilistic in nature.
K. Family history of mood disorder or suicide is common.

# Manic Episodes

I. **DSM-IV Diagnostic Criteria**
    A. At least one week of abnormally and persistently elevated, expansive or irritable mood (may be less than one week if hospitalization is required).
    B. During the period of mood disturbance, at least three of the following have persisted in a significant manner (four if mood is irritable):
       1. Inflated self-esteem or grandiosity.
       2. Decreased need for sleep.
       3. The patient has been more talkative than usual or feels pressure to keep talking.
       4. Flight of ideas (jumping from topic to topic) or a subjective sense of racing thoughts.
       5. Distractibility.
       6. Increased goal-directed activity or psychomotor agitation.
       7. Excessive involvement in pleasurable activities with a high potential for painful consequences (ie, sexual indiscretion).
    C. Does not meet criteria for a mixed episode.
    D. Symptoms must have cause marked impairment in social or occupational functioning, or have required hospitalization to prevent harm to self or others, or psychotic features are present.
    E. The symptoms cannot be caused by a medical condition, medication or drugs.
II. **Clinical Features of Manic Episodes**
    A. The most common presentation is excessive euphoria, but some patients may present with irritability alone.
    B. Patients may seek out constant enthusiastic interaction with others, frequently using poor judgment in those interactions.
    C. Increased psychomotor activity can take the form of excessive planning and participation, which are ultimately nonproductive.
    D. Reckless behavior with negative consequences is common (eg, shopping sprees, excessive spending, sexual promiscuity).
    E. Inability to sleep can be severe and persist for days.
    F. Lability of mood is common.
    G. Grandiose delusions are common.
    H. Speech is pressured, loud and intrusive, and difficulty interrupting these patients is common. Flight of ideas can result in gross disorganization and incoherence of speech.
    I. Patients frequently lack insight into their behavior and resist treatment.
    J. Patients may become grossly psychotic, most frequently with paranoid features.

**K.** Patients may become assaultive, particularly if psychotic.
**L.** Dysphoria is common at the height of a manic episode, and the patient may become suicidal.

# Hypomanic Episodes

I. **DSM-IV Diagnostic Criteria**
   **A.** At least 4 days of abnormally and persistently elevated, expansive or irritable mood.
   **B.** During the period of mood disturbance at least three of the following have persisted in a significant manner (four if mood is irritable):
      1. Inflated self-esteem or grandiosity.
      2. Decreased need for sleep.
      3. The patient is more talkative than usual and feels pressure to keep talking.
      4. Flight of ideas (jumping from topic to topic) or a subjective sense of racing thoughts.
      5. Distractibility.
      6. Increased goal-directed activity or psychomotor agitation.
      7. Excessive involvement in pleasurable activities that have a high potential for painful consequences (ie, sexual promiscuity).
   **C.** The mood disturbance and change in functioning is noticeable to others.
   **D.** The change in functioning is uncharacteristic of the patient's baseline but does not cause marked social or occupational dysfunction, does not require hospitalization, and no psychotic features are present.
   **E.** Symptoms cannot be due to a medical condition, medication or drugs.
II. **Clinical Features of Hypomanic Episodes**
   **A.** The major difference between hypomanic and manic episodes is the lack of major social and/or occupational dysfunction in hypomania, which is hallmark of a manic episode. Hallucinations and delusions are not seen in hypomania.

# Mixed Mood Episodes

I. **DSM-IV Diagnostic Criteria**
   **A.** Patient meets criteria for both for at least one week.
   **B.** Symptoms are severe enough to cause marked impairment in occupational or social functioning, require hospitalization, or psychotic features are present.
   **C.** Organic factors have been excluded (medical conditions, medications, drugs).
II. **Clinical Features of Mixed Mood Episodes**
   **A.** Patients subjectively experience rapidly shifting moods.
   **B.** They frequently present with agitation, psychosis, suicidality, appetite disturbance and insomnia.

# Major Depressive Disorder

**I. DSM-IV Diagnostic Criteria for Major Depressive Disorders**
   **A.** History of one or more Major Depressive Episodes.
   **B.** No history of manic, hypomanic, or mixed episodes.

**II. Clinical Features of Major Depressive Disorder**
   **A.** Major depressive disorder has a high mortality; 15% suicide rate. Common coexisting diagnoses include panic disorder, eating disorders, substance-related disorders. These disorders should be excluded by the clinical history.
   **B.** Major depressive disorder often complicates the presentation and treatment of patients with medical conditions, such as myocardial infarction, stroke, and diabetes.
   **C.** The disorder often follows an episode of severe stress, such as loss of a loved one.
   **D.** All patients should be asked about suicidal ideation as well as intent. Hospitalization may be necessary for acutely suicidal patients. Suicide risk may increase as the patient begins to respond to treatment. Lack of initiative and poor energy can improve prior to improvement in mood, allowing patients to follow through on suicidal ideas.
   **E.** Suicide risk is most closely related to the degree of hopelessness a patient is experiencing and not to the severity of depression.

**III. Epidemiology of Major Depressive Disorder**
   **A.** Prevalence is approximately 3-6%, with a 2:1 female-to-male ratio.
   **B.** Approximately 50% of patients who have a single episode of major depressive disorder will have a recurrence. This rises to 70% after two episodes and 90% after three episodes.
   **C.** Functioning returns to the premorbid level between episodes in approximately two-thirds of patients.
   **D.** The disorder is two times more common in first-degree relatives of patients with major depressive disorder compared to the general population.

**IV. Classification of Major Depressive Disorder**
   **A. Major Depressive Disorder with Psychotic Features.** Depression is accompanied by hallucinations or delusions, which may be mood-congruent (content is consistent with typical depressive themes) or mood incongruent (content does not involve typical depressive themes).
   **B. Major Depressive Disorder, Chronic.** Full diagnostic criteria for major depressive disorder have been met continuously for at least 2 years.
   **C. Major Depressive Disorder with Catatonic Features**
   **Accompanied by at least two of the following:**
      **1.** Motor immobility or stupor.
      **2.** Excessive purposeless motor activity.
      **3.** Extreme negativism or mutism.
      **4.** Bizarre or inappropriate posturing, stereotyped movement, or facial grimacing.
      **5.** Echolalia or echopraxia.
   **D. Major Depressive Disorder with Melancholic Features.** Depression is accompanied by severe anhedonia or lack of reactivity to usually pleasurable stimuli and at least three of the following:
      **1.** Quality of mood is distinctly depressed.
      **2.** Mood is worse in the morning.

  3. Early morning awakening.
  4. Marked psychomotor slowing.
  5. Significant weight loss.
  6. Excessive guilt.
- **E. Major Depressive Disorder with Atypical Features.** Depression is accompanied by mood reactivity and at least two of the following:
  1. Significant weight gain.
  2. Hypersomnia.
  3. "Heavy" feeling in extremities (leaden paralysis).
  4. Chronic pattern of rejection sensitivity, resulting in significant social or occupational dysfunction.
  5. Does not meet criteria for major depressive disorder with melancholic or catatonic features.
- **F. Major Depressive Disorder with Postpartum Onset.** Onset of episode within four weeks of parturition.
- **G. Major Depressive Disorder with Seasonal Pattern**
  1. Recurrent episodes of depression with a pattern of onset at same time each year.
  2. Full remissions occur at a characteristic time of year.
  3. Over a two-year period, at least two seasonal episodes have occurred, and no nonseasonal episodes have occurred.
  4. Seasonal episodes outnumber non-seasonal episodes.

## V. Differential Diagnosis of Major Depressive Disorder
### A. Bereavement
  1. Bereavement may share many symptoms of a major depressive episode.
  2. Normal bereavement should not present with depressive symptoms, which cause severe functional impairment lasting more than two months.
### B. Adjustment Disorder with Depressed Mood
  1. A stressful event may precede the onset of a major depressive episode; however, dysphoria related to a stressor that does not meet the criteria for major depressive episode should be diagnosed as an adjustment disorder.
### C. Anxiety Disorders
  1. Symptoms of anxiety frequently coexist with depression.
  2. When anxiety symptoms coexist with depressive symptoms, the depression should be the focus of treatment because it carries a higher morbidity and mortality. Antidepressants are often effective in treating anxiety disorders.
### D. Schizophrenia and Schizoaffective Disorder
  1. Subjective depression may accompany acute psychosis. Severe psychotic depression may be difficult to distinguish from a primary psychotic disorder.
  2. In psychotic depression, the mood symptoms generally precede the onset of psychotic symptoms.
  3. The premorbid and inter-episode functioning are generally higher in patients with mood disorders, compared to patients with psychotic disorders.

**E. Dementia**
1. Dementia and depression may present with complaints of apathy, poor concentration, and impaired memory.
2. Cognitive deficits due to a mood disorder may appear very similar to dementia. "Pseudodementia" is defined as depression that mimics dementia.
3. Differentiation of dementia from depression can be very difficult in the elderly. When the diagnosis is unclear, a trial of antidepressants may be useful because depression is reversible and dementia is not.
4. The medical history and examination can suggest possible medical or organic causes of dementia.

**F. Mood Disorder Due to a General Medical Condition**
1. The medical history and examination may suggest potential medical conditions which present with depressive symptoms.
2. This diagnosis applies when the mood disorder is a direct physiological consequence of the medical disorder and is not an emotional response to a physical illness. For example, Parkinson's disease is often associated with a depressive syndrome, which is not simply a reaction to the disability of the disease.

**G. Substance-Induced Mood Disorder**
1. Careful examination of all medications, drugs of abuse, or toxin exposure should be completed.
2. Alcohol, drug abuse, sedatives, antihypertensives, and oral contraceptives can all cause depressive symptoms.
3. Withdrawal from sympathomimetics or amphetamines may cause a depressive syndrome.

**VI. Pharmacotherapy of Depression**
**A.** For a complete discussion of the treatment of Depression, see Antidepressant Therapy, page 105.
**B. Selecting an Antidepressant Agent**
1. All antidepressant drugs have shown equal efficacy, but the various agents have different side-effect profiles.
2. There is no reliable method of predicting which patients will respond to a specific antidepressant based on clinical presentation. If the patient or a first-degree relative has had a previous treatment response to a given medication, another trial of that medication is indicated.
3. Agent selection is also based on the expected tolerance to side effects, the patient's age, suicide potential, and any coexisting diseases or medications.
   a. Selective-serotonin reuptake inhibitors (SSRIs) are much safer than heterocyclic antidepressants in patients with a history of cardiac disease.
   b. SSRIs are safer than heterocyclic antidepressants in overdose, making them preferable for suicidal patients.

**C. Classification of Antidepressant Agents**
1. **Heterocyclic Antidepressants**
   a. Side effects (especially sedation and anticholinergic effects) are worse during the first month of therapy and usually diminish after four weeks.
   b. Early in the treatment course, patients may sleep better, but patients rarely describe improvement in mood before 3-4 weeks.
   c. The potential of tricyclics to be fatal in overdose limits the quantity that should be prescribed, particularly in patients with suicidal

       ideation or a history of suicide attempts.

    **d.** Use of heterocyclic antidepressants in the elderly may be limited by the sensitivity of these patients to anticholinergic and cardio-vascular side effects.

## 2. Selective-Serotonin Reuptake Inhibitors (SSRIs)

    **a.** SSRIs are first-line agents and include fluoxetine (Prozac), sertraline (Zoloft), paroxetine (Paxil), fluvoxamine (Luvox), cita-lopram (Celexa), and escitalopram (Lexapro).

    **b.** SSRIs, with their comparatively benign side-effect profile, allow once-daily dosing and present less danger from overdose because they have reduced seizure potential and lack the cardiovascular toxicity of the tricyclics in overdose.

    **c.** Another advantage of SSRIs is that they require less dosage titration. Thus, a therapeutic dose may be achieved earlier than with tricyclics.

    **d.** Although many patients take SSRIs with no adverse consequences, the most frequent side effects are insomnia, headache, GI upset, anxiety, agitation, and sexual dysfunction.

## 3. Atypical Agents

    **a. Bupropion (Wellbutrin, Wellbutrin SR, and Wellbutrin XL):** Bupropion is a mildly stimulating antidepressant and is particularly useful in patients who have had sexual impairment from other drugs. The short half-life of bupropion requires multiple daily doses, complicating compliance. There is a low incidence of sexual dysfunction and possible decreased liability to precipitate mania.

    **b. Venlafaxine (Effexor, Effexor XR):** Venlafaxine is a selective inhibitor of serotonin reuptake with norepinephrine reuptake inhibition occurring at doses > 200 mg/day. Insomnia, nervousness and nausea are common. At higher doses, it can elevate diastolic blood pressure and requires monitoring of blood pressure.

    **c. Nefazodone:** Nefazodone is a serotonergic antidepressant, but it is not considered a SSRI because of other receptor effects. It tends to be more sedating than the SSRIs, and it can have a calming or antianxiety effect in some patients. It is also useful in patients who experience sexual impairment with other antidepressants. Rare cases of liver failure have been reported with nefazodone (one case of death or liver transplant per 250,000-300,000 patient-years of nefazodone exposure).

    **d. Mirtazapine (Remeron):** Mirtazapine is a selective alpha-2-adrenergic antagonist, which enhances noradrenergic and serotonergic neurotransmission. Sedation and enhanced appetite are inversely proportional to dose, prompting some clinicians to forgo dose titration. There is a low incidence of sexual dysfunction.

    **e. Duloxetine (Cymbalta):** Duloxetine is a norepinephrine and serotonin reuptake inhibitor at all doses. It is indicated for major depression and neuropathic pain. Most common side effects include nausea, and insomnia.

## 4. Monoamine Oxidase Inhibitors (MAOIs)

    **a.** Contraindications and dietary restriction discourage common use.

    **b. Side Effects.** Orthostatic hypotension is common. A tyramine-free diet is required to prevent hypertensive crisis.

    **c. Drug Interactions.** Coadministration of epinephrine, meperidine (Demerol), and SSRIs can be life-threatening.

VII. **Electroconvulsive Therapy for Depression** (also see Electroconvulsive Therapy, page 118). ECT is a safe and very effective treatment for depression, especially if there is a high risk for suicide or insufficient time for a trial of medication.

VIII. **Psychotherapy for Major Depressive Disorder**
   A. A wide variety of psychotherapies are effective in the treatment of major depressive disorder, especially cognitive behavioral psychotherapy and insight oriented psychotherapy.
   B. Combined pharmacotherapy and psychotherapy is the most effective treatment for major depressive disorder, after ETC.

# Dysthymic Disorder

I. **DSM-IV Diagnostic Criteria**
   A. Depressed mood is present for most of the day, for more days than it is not present, and depression has been present for at least two years.
   B. **Presence of at least two of the following:**
      1. Poor appetite or overeating.
      2. Insomnia or hypersomnia.
      3. Low energy or fatigue.
      4. Low self-esteem.
      5. Poor concentration or difficulty making decisions.
      6. Hopelessness.
   C. Over the two-year period, the patient has never been without symptoms for more than two months consecutively.
   D. No major depressive episode has occurred during the first two years of the disturbance.
   E. No manic, hypomanic or mixed episode, or evidence of cyclothymia is present.
   F. Symptoms do not occur with a chronic psychotic disorder.
   G. Symptoms are not due to substance use or a general medical condition.
   H. Symptoms cause significant social or occupational dysfunction or marked subjective distress.

II. **Clinical Features of Dysthymic Disorder**
   A. Symptoms of dysthymic disorder are similar to those of major depression. The most common symptoms are loss of pleasure in usually pleasurable activities, feelings of inadequacy, social withdrawal, guilt, irritability, and decreased productivity.
   B. Changes in sleep, appetite or psychomotor behavior are less common than in major depressive disorder.
   C. Patients often complain of multiple physical problems, which may interfere with occupational or social functioning. Psychotic symptoms are not present.
   D. Episodes of major depression may occur after the first two years of the disorder. The combination of dysthymia and major depression is known as "double depression."

III. **Epidemiology of Dysthymic Disorder**
   A. Lifetime prevalence is 6%, with a female-to-male ratio of 3:1.
   B. Onset usually occurs in childhood or adolescence.
   C. Dysthymia that occurs prior to the onset of major depression has a worse prognosis than major depression without dysthymia.

**IV. Classification of Dysthymic Disorder**
  A. **Early Onset Dysthymia:** Onset occurs before age 21.
  B. **Late Onset Dysthymia:** Onset occurs at age 21 or older.
  C. Dysthymia with Atypical Features is accompanied by mood reactivity and at least two of the following:
    1. Significant weight gain.
    2. Hypersomnia.
    3. "Leaden" paralysis, characterized by a feeling of being heavy or weighted down physically.
    4. A chronic pattern of rejection sensitivity, which often results in significant social or occupational dysfunction.

**V. Differential Diagnosis of Dysthymic Disorder**
  A. **Major Depressive Disorder.** Dysthymia leads to chronic, less severe depressive symptoms, compared to Major Depression. Major Depression usually has one of more discrete episodes.
  B. **Substance-Induced Mood Disorder.** Alcohol, benzodiazepines and other sedative-hypnotics can mimic dysthymia symptoms, as can chronic use of amphetamines or cocaine. Anabolic steroids, oral contraceptives, methyldopa, beta-adrenergic blockers and isotretinoin (Accutane) have also been linked to depressive symptoms. Substance-Induced Mood Disorder should be excluded with a careful history of drugs of abuse and medications.
  C. **Mood Disorder Due to a General Medical Condition.** Depressive symptoms consistent with dysthymia may occur in stroke, Parkinson's disease, multiple sclerosis, Huntington's disease, vitamin $B_{12}$ deficiency, hypothyroidism, Cushing's disease, pancreatic carcinoma, and HIV. These disorders should be ruled out with a history, physical examination, and labs as indicated.
  D. **Psychotic Disorders.** Depressive symptoms are common in chronic psychotic disorders, and dysthymia should not be diagnosed if symptoms occur only during psychosis.
  E. **Personality Disorders.** Personality disorders frequently coexist with dysthymic disorder.

**VI. Treatment of Dysthymic Disorder**
  A. Hospitalization is usually not required unless suicidality is present.
  B. **Antidepressants**. Many patients respond well to antidepressants. SSRIs are most often used. If these or other antidepressants, such as venlafaxine, nefazodone or bupropion, have failed, then a tricyclic antidepressant, such as desipramine, 150 to 200 mg per day, is often effective. (For a complete discussion of antidepressant therapy, see page 105.)
  C. **Psychotherapy:** Cognitive psychotherapy may help patients deal with incorrect negative attitudes about themselves. Insight oriented psychotherapy may help patients resolve early childhood conflict, which may have precipitated depressive symptoms. Combined psychotherapy and pharmacotherapy produces the best outcome.

# Bipolar I Disorder

Bipolar I Disorder is a disorder in which at least one manic or mixed episode is present.

## I. DSM-IV Criteria for Bipolar I Disorder
   A. One or more manic or mixed episodes.
   B. The disorder is commonly accompanied by a history of one or more major depressive episodes, but a major depressive episode is not required for the diagnosis.
   C. Manic or mixed episodes cannot be due to a medical condition, medication, drugs of abuse, toxins, or treatment for depression.
   D. Symptoms cannot be caused by a psychotic disorder.

## II. Clinical Features of Bipolar I Disorder
   A. The first mood episode in bipolar disorder is often depression, especially in women.
   B. Ninety percent of patients who have a single manic episode will have a recurrence.
   C. Bipolar disorder is often diagnosed over time. Studies find that 10 years may elapse between the first mood episode and the diagnosis of bipolar.
   D. Episodes occur more frequently with age.
   E. Manic episodes can result in violence, child abuse, excessive debt, job loss, or divorce.
   F. Mixed episodes are more likely in younger patients.
   G. The suicide rate of bipolar patients is 10-15%.
   H. Common comorbid diagnoses often include substance-related disorders, eating disorders, and attention deficit hyperactivity disorder.
   I. Bipolar I disorder with a rapid cycling pattern carries a poor prognosis and may affect up to 20% of bipolar patients.
   J. A thorough past psychiatric and family history is essential when evaluating a patient with mood disorder.

## III. Epidemiology of Bipolar I Disorder
   A. The lifetime prevalence of bipolar disorder is approximately 0.5-1.5%.
   B. The male-to-female ratio is 1:1
   C. The first episode in males tends to be a manic episode, while the first episode in females tends to be a depressive episode.
   D. First-degree relatives have higher rates of mood disorder. Bipolar disorder has a 70% concordance rate among monozygotic twins.

## IV. Classification of Bipolar I Disorder
   A. Classification of bipolar I disorder involves describing the current or most recent mood episode as either manic, hypomanic, mixed or depressive (eg, Bipolar I disorder- most recent episode mixed).
   B. **The most recent episode can be further classified as follows:**
      1. Without psychotic features.
      2. With psychotic features.
      3. With catatonic features.
      4. With postpartum onset.
   C. **Bipolar I Disorder with Rapid Cycling**
      1. Diagnosis requires the presence of at least four mood episodes within one year.
      2. Rapid cycling mood episodes may include major depressive, manic, hypomanic, or mixed episodes

**3.** The patient must be symptom-free for at least two months between episodes, or the patient must switch to an opposite episode.

## V. Differential Diagnosis of Bipolar I Disorder

**A. Cyclothymic Disorder.** This disorder may cause manic-like episodes that do not meet the criteria for manic episode, depressive episodes, or major depression.

**B. Psychotic Disorders**

  **1.** The clinical presentation of a patient at the height of a manic episode may be indistinguishable from that of an acute exacerbation of paranoid schizophrenia.

  **2.** If the history is unavailable or if the patient is having an initial episode, it may be necessary to observe the patient over time to make an accurate diagnosis. A subsequent major depressive episode or manic episode that initially presents with mood symptoms prior to the onset of psychosis, indicates that a mood disorder, rather than a psychotic disorder, is present.

  **3.** A family history of either a mood disorder or psychotic disorder suggests the diagnosis of bipolar disorder or psychotic disorder, respectively.

**C. Substance-Induced Mood Disorder.** The effects of medication or drugs of abuse should be excluded. Common organic causes of mania include sympathomimetics, amphetamines, cocaine, steroids, and $H_2$ blockers (eg, cimetidine).

**D. Mood Disorder Due to a General Medical Condition.** Medical conditions that may present with manic symptoms include AIDS, Cushing's, hyperthyroidism, lupus, multiple sclerosis, and brain tumors.

## VI. Treatment of Bipolar I Disorder

**A.** Hospitalization may be necessary for either Manic or Depressive mood episodes.

**B.** Assessment of suicidality is essential; suicidal ideation and intent should be evaluated. Medications reduce the incidence of suicide in bipolar disorder.

**C. Pharmacotherapy**

  **1.** Traditional mood stabilizers, such as lithium and the anticonvulsants, are effective for acute treatment as well as the prophylaxis of mood episodes. (Also see Mood Stabilizers, page 110). Mood stabilizers are more effective in preventing and treating manic episodes than they are for depressive episodes. Lamotrigine is modestly effective in treating bipolar depression, but more so than lithium and other anticonvulsants.

  **2.** Antidepressants may be used for treatment of major depressive episodes, but they should only be used in conjunction with a mood stabilizer to prevent precipitation of a manic episode. Tricyclics and serotonin-norepinephrine reuptake inhibitors (venlafaxine and duloxetine) may have higher risk for precipitating mania. Antidepressants may induce rapid cycling.

  **3.** All atypical antipsychotics are effective in acute mania. Aripiprazole and olanzapine are approved for maintenance treatment and data are accumulating that other atypicals are effective as well for long-term use. The combination medication olanzapine-fluoxetine is approved for treatment of bipolar depression.

  **4.** Sedating benzodiazepines, such as clonazepam and lorazepam, may be used adjunctively for severe agitation associated with acute mania.

  **5.** ECT is very effective for bipolar disorder (depressed or manic episodes), but it is generally used after conventional pharmacotherapy has failed or is contraindicated.

**D. Psychotherapy**
1. Therapy aimed at increasing insight and dealing with the consequences of the manic episodes may be very helpful.
2. Family or marital therapy may also help increase understanding and tolerance of the affected family member.

# Bipolar II Disorder

**I. DSM-IV Diagnostic Criteria of Bipolar II Disorder**
  A. One or more major depressive episodes and at least one hypomanic episode.
  B. Mood episodes cannot be caused by a medical condition, medication, drugs of abuse, toxins, or treatment for depression.
  C. Symptoms cannot be caused by a psychotic disorder.

**II. Clinical Features of Bipolar II Disorder**
  A. Hypomanic episodes tend to occur in close proximity to depressive episodes, and episodes tend to occur more frequently with age.
  B. Social and occupational consequences of bipolar II can include job loss and divorce. These patients have a suicide rate of 10-15%.
  C. Common comorbid diagnoses include substance-related disorders, eating disorders, attention deficit hyperactivity disorder, and borderline personality disorder.
  D. The rapid cycling pattern carries a poor prognosis.

**III. Epidemiology.** The lifetime prevalence of bipolar II is 0.5%. It is more common in women than in men.

**IV. Classification of Bipolar II Disorder**
  A. Classification of bipolar II disorder involves evaluation of current or most recent mood episode, which can be hypomanic or depressive.
  **B. The most recent episode can be further classified as follows:**
   1. Episodes without psychotic features.
   2. Episodes with psychotic features.
   3. Episodes with catatonic features.
   4. Episodes with post partum onset.
  **C. Bipolar II Disorder with Rapid Cycling**
   1. This diagnosis requires the presence of at least four mood episodes within one year. Episodes may include major depressive, manic, hypomanic, or mixed type episodes.
   2. The patient must be symptom-free for at least two months between episodes, or the patient must display a change in mood to an opposite type of episode.

**V. Differential Diagnosis of Bipolar II Disorder**
  A. **Cyclothymic Disorder.** These patients will exhibit mood swings that do not meet the criteria for full manic episode or full major depressive episode.
  B. **Substance-Induced Mood Disorder.** The effects of medication, drugs of abuse, or toxin exposure should be excluded.
  C. **Mood Disorder Due to a General Medical Condition.** Manic symptoms can be associated with AIDS, Cushing's, hyperthyroidism, lupus, multiple sclerosis, and brain tumors. Depressive symptoms consistent with

dysthymia may occur in stroke, Parkinson's disease, multiple sclerosis, Huntington's disease, vitamin $B_{12}$ deficiency, hypothyroidism, Cushing's disease, pancreatic carcinoma, and HIV.

**VI.Treatment of Bipolar II Disorder.** The treatment of Bipolar II disorder includes a mood stabilizer and an antidepressant if depression is present. Treatment is similar to that of Bipolar I disorder, described above (See Mood Stabilizers, page 110).

# Cyclothymic Disorder

Cyclothymic disorder consists of chronic cyclical episodes of mild depression and symptoms of mild mania.

**I. DSM-IV Diagnostic Criteria**
   **A.** Many periods of depression and hypomania, occurring for at least two years. Depressive episodes do not reach the severity of major depression.
   **B.** During the two-year period, the patient has not been symptom-free for more than two months at a time.
   **C.** During the two-year period, no episodes of major depression, mania or mixed states were present.
   **D.** Symptoms are not accounted for by schizoaffective disorder and do not coexist with schizophrenia, schizophreniform disorder, delusional disorder, or any other psychotic disorder.
   **E.** Symptoms are not caused by substance use or a general medical condition.
   **F.** Symptoms cause significant distress or functional impairment.

**II. Clinical Features of Cyclothymic Disorder**
   **A.** Symptoms are similar to those of bipolar I disorder, but they are of a lesser magnitude and cycles occur at a faster rate.
   **B.** Patients frequently have coexisting substance abuse.
   **C.** One-third of patients develop a severe mood disorder (usually bipolar II).
   **D.** Occupational and interpersonal impairment is frequent and usually a consequence of hypomanic states.
   **E.** Cyclothymic disorder often coexists with borderline personality disorder.

**III. Epidemiology of Cyclothymic Disorder**
   **A.** The prevalence is 1%, but cyclothymic disorder constitutes 5-10% of psychiatric outpatients.
   **B.** The onset occurs between age 15 and 25, and women are affected more than men by a ratio of 3:2.
   **C.** Thirty percent of patients have a family history of bipolar disorder.

**IV. Differential Diagnosis of Cyclothymic Disorder**
   **A. Bipolar II Disorder.** Patients with bipolar type II disorder exhibit hypomania and episodes of major depression.
   **B. Substance-Induced Mood Disorder/Mood Disorder Due to a General Medical Condition.** Hypomanic symptoms can be associated with AIDS, Cushing's, hyperthyroidism, lupus, multiple sclerosis, and brain tumors. Depressive symptoms consistent with dysthymia may occur in stroke, Parkinson's disease, multiple sclerosis, Huntington's disease, vitamin $B_{12}$ deficiency, hypothyroidism, Cushing's disease, pancreatic carcinoma, and HIV.
   **C. Personality Disorders** (antisocial, borderline, histrionic, narcissistic) can

be associated with marked shifts in mood. Personality disorders may coexist with cyclothymic disorder.

## V. Treatment of Cyclothymic Disorder

**A.** Mood stabilizers are the treatment of choice, and lithium is effective in 60% of patients. The clinical use of mood stabilizers is similar to that of bipolar disorder. (Also see Mood Stabilizers, page 110).

**B.** Depressive episodes must be treated cautiously because of the risk of precipitating manic symptoms with antidepressants (occurs in 50% of patients) or increase the rate of cycling. The serotonin-norepinephrine re-uptake inhibitors and tricyclics may have greater risk. A conservative approach would be to treat concurrently with an antidepressant and a mood stabilizer.

**C.** Patients often require supportive therapy to improve awareness of their illness and to deal with the functional consequences of their behavior.

### References
References, see page 120.

# *Anxiety Disorders*

## Generalized Anxiety Disorder

Generalized anxiety disorder (GAD) is the most common of the anxiety disorders. It is characterized by unrealistic or excessive anxiety and worry about two or more life circumstances for at least six months.

I. **DSM-IV Diagnostic Criteria for Generalized Anxiety Disorder**
   A. Excessive anxiety or worry is present most days during at least a six-month period and involves a number of life events.
   B. The anxiety is difficult to control.
   C. **At least three of the following:**
      1. Restlessness or feeling on edge.
      2. Easy fatigability.
      3. Difficulty concentrating.
      4. Irritability.
      5. Muscle tension.
      6. Sleep disturbance.
   D. The focus of anxiety is not anticipatory anxiety about having a panic attack, as in panic disorder.
   E. The anxiety or physical symptoms cause significant distress or impairment in functioning.
   F. Symptoms are not caused by substance use or a medical condition, and symptoms are not related to a mood or psychotic disorder.

II. **Clinical Features of Generalized Anxiety Disorder**
   A. Other features often include insomnia, irritability, trembling, muscle aches and soreness, muscle twitches, clammy hands, dry mouth, and a heightened startle reflex. Patients may also report palpitations, dizziness, difficulty breathing, urinary frequency, dysphagia, light-headedness, abdominal pain, and diarrhea.
   B. Patients often complain that they "can't stop worrying," which may revolve around valid concerns about money, jobs, marriage, health, and the safety of children.
   C. Chronic worry is a prominent feature of generalized anxiety disorder, unlike the intermittent terror that characterizes panic disorder.
   D. Mood disorders, substance- and stress-related disorders (headaches, dyspepsia) commonly coexist with GAD. Up to one-fourth of GAD patients develop panic disorder. Excessive worry and somatic symptoms, including autonomic hyperactivity and hypervigilance, occur most days.
   E. About 30-50% of patients with anxiety disorders will also meet criteria for major depressive disorder. Drugs and alcohol may cause anxiety or may be an attempt at self-treatment. Substance abuse may be a complication of GAD.

III. **Epidemiology**
   A. Lifetime prevalence is 5%.
   B. The female-to-male sex ratio for GAD is 2:1.
   C. Most patients report excessive anxiety during childhood or adolescence; however, onset after age 20 may sometimes occur.

## IV. Differential Diagnosis of Generalized Anxiety Disorder

**A. Substance-Induced Anxiety Disorder.** Substances such as caffeine, amphetamines, or cocaine can cause anxiety symptoms. Alcohol or benzodiazepine withdrawal can mimic symptoms of GAD. These disorders should be excluded by history and toxicology screen.

**B. Panic Disorder, Obsessive-Compulsive Disorder, Social Phobia, Hypochondriasis and Anorexia Nervosa**
1. Many psychiatric disorders present with marked anxiety, and the diagnosis of GAD should be made only if the anxiety is unrelated to the other disorders.
2. For example, GAD should not be diagnosed in panic disorder if the patient has excessive anxiety about having a panic attack, or if an anorexic patient has anxiety about weight gain.

**C. Anxiety Disorder Due to a General Medical Condition.** Hyperthyroidism, cardiac arrhythmias, pulmonary embolism, congestive heart failure, and hypoglycemia, may produce significant anxiety and should be ruled out as clinically indicated.

**D. Mood and Psychotic Disorders**
1. Excessive worry and anxiety occurs in many mood and psychotic disorders.
2. If anxiety occurs only during the course of the mood or psychotic disorder, then GAD cannot be diagnosed.

## V. Laboratory Evaluation of Anxiety

**A.** Serum glucose, calcium and phosphate levels, electrocardiogram, and thyroid studies should be included in the initial workup of all patients.

**B. Other Studies.** Urine drug screen and urinary catecholamine levels may be required to exclude specific disorders.

## VI. Treatment of Generalized Anxiety Disorder

**A.** The combination of pharmacologic therapy and psychotherapy is the most successful form of treatment.

## VII. Pharmacotherapy of Generalized Anxiety Disorder

**A. Antidepressants**
1. **SSRIs** and Venlafaxine (Effexor and Effexor XR) are first-line treatments for GAD. Effexor XR can be started at 75 mg per day; however, patients with severe anxiety or panic attacks should begin at 37.5 mg per day. The dose should then be titrated up to a maximum dosage of 225 mg of Effexor XR per day.
2. The onset of action of antidepressants is much slower than the benzodiazepines, but they have no addictive potential and may be more effective. An antidepressant is the agent of choice when depression coexists with anxiety.
3. The side-effect profile for GAD patients is similar to that seen with depressive disorders.
4. Tricyclic antidepressants are also effective in treating GAD, but adverse effects limit their use.
5. **Buspirone (BuSpar)**
   a. Buspirone is an effective treatment for GAD. Buspirone usually requires 3-6 weeks at a dosage of 10-20 mg tid for efficacy. It lacks sedative effects. Tolerance to the beneficial effects of buspirone does not seem to develop. There is no physiologic dependence or withdrawal syndrome.
   b. Combined benzodiazepine-buspirone therapy may be used for generalized anxiety disorder, with subsequent tapering of the

benzodiazepine after 2-4 weeks.
   c. Patients who have been previously treated with benzodiazepines or who have a history of substance abuse have a decreased response to buspirone.
   d. Buspirone may have some antidepressant effects.

## B. Benzodiazepines
   1. Benzodiazepines can almost always relieve anxiety if given in adequate doses, and they have no delayed onset of action.
   2. Long-term use of benzodiazepines should be reserved for patients who have failed to respond to venlafaxine (Effexor), SSRIs, buspirone (BuSpar) and other antidepressants, or who are intolerant to their side effects.
   3. Benzodiazepines are very useful for treating anxiety during the period in which it takes buspirone or antidepressants to exert their effects. Benzodiazepines should then be tapered after several weeks.
   4. Benzodiazepines have few side effects other than sedation. Tolerance to their sedative effects develops but not to their antianxiety properties.
   5. Since clonazepam (Klonopin) and diazepam (Valium) have long half-lives, they are less likely to result in interdose anxiety and are easier to taper.
   6. Drug dependency becomes a clinical issue if the benzodiazepine is used regularly for more than 2-3 weeks. A withdrawal syndrome occurs in 70% of patients, characterized by intense anxiety, tremulousness dysphoria, sleep and perceptual disturbances and appetite suppression. Slow tapering of benzodiazepines is crucial (especially those with short half-lives).

## C. Non-Drug Approaches to Anxiety
   1. Patients should stop drinking coffee and other caffeinated beverages, and avoid excessive alcohol consumption.
   2. Patients should get adequate sleep, with the use of medication if necessary. Moderate exercise each day may help reduce the intensity of anxiety symptoms.
   3. Psychotherapy
      a. Cognitive behavioral therapy, with emphasis on relaxation techniques and instruction on misinterpretation of physiologic symptoms, may improve functioning in mild cases.
      b. Supportive or insight oriented psychotherapy can be helpful in mild cases of anxiety.

# Panic Disorder

Patients with panic disorder report discrete periods of intense terror and fear of impending doom, which are almost intolerable.

## I. DSM-IV Criteria for Panic Disorder with Agoraphobia
### A. Both 1 and 2 are Required
   1. Recurrent unexpected panic attacks occur, during which four of the following symptoms begin abruptly and reach a peak within 10 minutes in the presence of intense fear:
      a. Palpitations, increased heart rate.
      b. Sweating.

        **c.** Trembling or shaking.
        **d.** Sensation of shortness of breath.
        **e.** Feeling of choking.
        **f.** Chest pain or discomfort.
        **g.** Nausea or abdominal distress.
        **h.** Feeling dizzy, lightheaded or faint.
        **i.** Derealization or depersonalization.
        **j.** Fear of losing control or going crazy.
        **k.** Fear of dying.
        **l.** Paresthesias.
        **m.** Chills or hot flushes.
    **2.** At least one of the attacks has been followed by one month of one of the following:
        **a.** Persistent concern about having additional attacks.
        **b.** Worry about the implications of the attack, such as fear of having a heart attack or going crazy.
        **c.** A significant change in behavior related to the attacks.
  **B.** The presence of agoraphobia has the following three components:
    **1.** Anxiety about being in places or situations where escape might be difficult or embarrassing, or in which help might not be available.
    **2.** Situations are avoided or endured with marked distress, or these situations are endured with anxiety about developing panic symptoms, or these situations require the presence of a companion.
    **3.** The anxiety is not better accounted for by another disorder, such as social phobia, where phobic avoidance is only limited to social situations.
  **C.** Panic attacks are not due to the effects of a substance or medical condition.
  **D.** The panic attacks are not caused by another mental disorder, such as panic on exposure to social situations in social phobia, or panic in response to stimuli of a severe stressor, such as with post-traumatic stress disorder.

**II. DSM-IV Criteria for Panic Disorder without Agoraphobia.** The DSM-IV diagnostic criteria are the same as panic disorder with agoraphobia, except there are no symptoms of agoraphobia.

**III. Clinical Features of Panic Disorder**
  **A.** Patients often believe that they have a serious medical condition. Marked anxiety about having future panic attacks (anticipatory anxiety) is common.
  **B.** In agoraphobia, the most common fears are of being outside alone or of being in crowds or traveling. The first panic attack often occurs without an acute stressor or warning. Later in the disorder, panic attacks may occur in relation to specific situations, and phobic avoidance to these situations can occur.
  **C.** Major Depression occurs in over fifty percent of patients. Agoraphobia may develop in patients with simple panic attacks. Elevation of blood pressure and tachycardia may occur during a panic attack.

**IV. Epidemiology of Panic Disorder**
  **A.** The lifetime prevalence of panic disorder is between 1.5% and 3.5%. The female-to-male ratio is 3:1. Up to one-half of panic disorder patients have agoraphobia.
  **B.** Panic disorder usually develops in early adulthood with a peak onset in

the mid twenties. Onset after age 45 years is unusual.
    C. First-degree relatives have an eightfold increase in panic disorder.
    D. The course of the illness is often chronic, but symptoms may wax and wane depending on the presence of stressors. Fifty percent of panic disorder patients are only mildly affected. Twenty percent have marked symptomatology.
    E. The suicide risk is markedly increased, especially in untreated patients. Substance abuse, especially of alcohol, may occur in up to 40% of patients.

## V. Classification of Panic Disorder
   A. **Unexpected Panic Attacks.** These panic attacks occur spontaneously without any situational trigger.
   B. **Situationally Bound Panic Attacks.** These panic attacks occur immediately after exposure to the feared stimulus, such as being in a high place or in an elevator.
   C. **Situationally Predisposed Panic Attacks.** These panic attacks usually occur upon exposure to the feared stimulus, but they do not necessarily occur immediately after every exposure. For example, an individual may have panic attacks in crowded situations, but he may not have an attack in every situation, or the attack may occur only after spending a significant amount of time in a crowded location.

## VI. Differential Diagnosis of Panic Disorder
   A. **Generalized Anxiety Disorder.** Anxiety is more constant than in panic disorder. Panic disorder is characterized by discrete episodes of severe anxiety along with physiologic symptoms.
   B. **Substance-Induced Anxiety Disorder.** Amphetamines, cocaine or caffeine can mimic panic attacks. Physiologic withdrawal from alcohol, benzodiazepines or barbiturates can also precipitate panic attacks.
   C. **Anxiety Due to a General Medical Condition.** Pheochromocytoma may mimic panic disorder and is characterized by markedly elevated blood pressure during the episodes of anxiety. It is excluded by a 24-hour urine assay for metanephrine or by serum catecholamines. Cardiac arrhythmias, hyperthyroidism, pulmonary embolism and hypoxia can present with symptoms similar to panic attacks.

## VII. Treatment of Panic Disorder
   A. Mild cases of panic disorder can be effectively treated with cognitive behavioral psychotherapy with an emphasis on relaxation and instruction on misinterpretation of physiologic symptoms.
   B. Pharmacotherapy is indicated when patients have marked distress from panic attacks or are experiencing impairment in work or social functioning.
      1. Serotonin-specific reuptake inhibitors and tricyclic antidepressants are most often used.
      2. SSRIs are the first-line treatment for panic disorder. Initiate treatment at lower doses than used in depression because routine antidepressant doses may actually increase anxiety in panic disorder patients. For example, 5-10 mg of paroxetine (Paxil) or 12.5-25 mg of sertraline (Zoloft) is used initially. The dose may then be gradually increased up to 20-40 mg for paroxetine or 50 to 100 mg for sertraline. Fluoxetine (Prozac) may exacerbate panic symptoms unless begun at very low doses (2-5 mg). Venlafaxine, citalopram, and escitalopram are also effective.
      3. When using a tricyclic antidepressant, the initial dose should also be low because of the potential for exacerbating panic symptoms early in

treatment. Imipramine (Tofranil) is the best studied agent, and it should be started at 10-25 mg per day, then increased slowly up to 100-200 mg per day as tolerated.

4. Benzodiazepines may be used adjunctively with TCAs or SSRIs during the first few weeks of treatment. When a patient has failed other agents, benzodiazepines are very effective. Alprazolam (Xanax) should be given four times a day to decrease interdose anxiety. The average dose is 0.5 mg qid (2 mg/day). Some patients may require up to 6 mg per day. A long-acting agent such as clonazepam (Klonopin) is also effective and causes less interdose anxiety compared to alprazolam. Clonazepam can be given less frequently than alprazolam.

5. Buspirone (BuSpar) is not effective for panic disorder.

6. Monoamine oxidase inhibitors(MAOIs) may be the most effective agents available for panic disorder, but these agents are not often used because of concern over hypertensive crisis.

7. Medication should be combined with cognitive-behavioral therapy for optimal outcome.

# Obsessive-Compulsive Disorder (OCD)

I. **DSM-IV Criteria for Obsessive-Compulsive Disorder**
   A. **Either Obsessions or Compulsions are present**
      1. **Obsessions**
         a. Recurrent, persistent thoughts, impulses, or images experienced as intrusive and causing marked anxiety.
         b. The thoughts, impulses, or images are not limited to excessive worries about real problems.
         c. The person attempts to ignore or suppress symptoms, or attempts to neutralize them with some other thought or action.
         d. The person recognizes the thoughts, impulses or images as a product of his or her own mind.
      2. **Compulsions**
         a. Repetitive behaviors or acts that the person feels driven to perform in response to an obsession.
         b. These behaviors or mental acts are aimed at preventing distress or preventing a specific dreaded event, but they are not connected in a realistic way to what they are attempting to prevent, or they are clearly excessive.
      3. The person has recognized that the obsessions or compulsions are excessive or unreasonable.
      4. The obsessions or compulsions cause marked distress, take more than a hour a day, or significantly interfere with functioning.
      5. If another psychiatric disorder is present, the content of the symptoms is not restricted to the disorder (eg, preoccupation with food in an eating disorder.
      6. The disturbance is not caused by substance abuse or a medical condition.
      7. Specify if the patient has poor insight into his illness. Poor insight is present if, for most of the current episode, the person does not recognize the symptoms as excessive or unreasonable.

## II. Clinical Features of Obsessive-Compulsive Disorder

**A.** Compulsions often occupy a large portion of an individuals day, leading to marked occupational and social impairment.

**B.** Situations that provoke symptoms are often avoided, such as when an individual with obsessions of contamination avoids touching anything that might be dirty.

**C.** Depression is common in patients with OCD. Alcohol or sedative-hypnotic drug abuse is common in patients with OCD because they attempt to use the drug to reduce distress.

**D.** Washing and checking rituals are common in children with OCD, and these children may not consider their behavior to be unreasonable or excessive.

**E.** Patients are reluctant to discuss symptoms, leading to an underdiagnosis of OCD.

## III. Epidemiology of Obsessive-Compulsive Disorder

**A.** The lifetime prevalence of OCD is approximately 2.5%. There is no sex difference in prevalence, but the age of onset is earlier in males.

**B.** The concordance rate for monozygotic twins is markedly higher compared to dizygotic twins.

**C.** OCD usually begins in adolescence or early adulthood, but it may occasionally begin in childhood.

**D.** The onset is usually gradual and most patients have a chronic disease course with waxing and waning of symptoms in relation to life stressors.

**E.** Fifteen percent of patients have a chronic debilitating course with marked impairment in social and occupational functioning.

**F.** Up to 50% of patients with Tourette's disorder have coexisting OCD; however, only 5% of OCD patients have Tourette's disorder.

## IV. Differential Diagnosis of Obsessive-Compulsive Disorder

**A. Substance-Induced Anxiety Disorder or Anxiety Disorder Due to a Medical Condition.** Amphetamines, cocaine, caffeine and other sympto-matic agents may mimic the anxiety symptoms of OCD. On rare occasions a brain tumor or temporal lobe epilepsy can manifest with OCD symptoms.

**B. Major Depressive Disorder.** Major depression may be associated with severe obsessive ruminations (eg, obsessive rumination about finances or a relationship). These obsessive thoughts are usually not associated with compulsive behaviors and are accompanied by other symptoms of depression.

**C. Generalized Anxiety Disorder.** In GAD, obsessive worries are about real life situations; however, in OCD, obsessions usually do not involve real life situations.

**D. Specific or Social Phobia, Body Dysmorphic Disorder or Trichotillo-mania.** Recurrent thoughts, behaviors or impulses may occur in these disorders. OCD should not be diagnosed if symptoms are caused by another psychiatric condition (eg, hair pulling in trichotillomania).

**E. Schizophrenia.** Patients with schizophrenia may have obsessive thoughts or compulsive behaviors; however, schizophrenia is associated with frank hallucinations and delusions.

**F. Obsessive-Compulsive Personality Disorder (OCPD).** Individuals with OCPD are preoccupied with perfectionism, order, and control, and they do not believe that their behavior is abnormal. They do not exhibit obsessions or compulsions.

## V. Treatment of Obsessive-Compulsive Disorder
   A. Pharmacotherapy is almost always indicated.
   B. Clomipramine (Anafranil), sertraline (Zoloft), paroxetine (Paxil) fluoxetine (Prozac), citalopram (Celexa), escitalopram (Lexapro) and fluvoxamine (Luvox) are effective.
   C. Standard antidepressant doses of clomipramine are usually effective, but higher doses of SSRIs are usually required, such as fluoxetine (Prozac) 60-80 mg, paroxetine (Paxil) 40-60 mg, or sertraline (Zoloft) 200 mg.
   D. Behavior therapy, such as cognitive-behavioral therapy, thought stopping, desensitization or flooding, may also be effective. A combination of behavioral therapy and medication is most effective.
   E. It is rare for treatment to completely eliminate the symptoms of OCD, but significant clinical improvement in symptoms can occur, and the patient's functioning can be drastically enhanced.

# Social Phobia

## I. DSM-IV Diagnostic Criteria for Social Phobia (also know as Social Anxiety Disorder)
   1. A marked and persistent fear of social or performance situations in which the person is exposed to unfamiliar people or to scrutiny by others. The individual often fears that he will act in a way that will be humiliating or embarrassing.
   2. Exposure to the feared situation almost invariably provokes anxiety, which may take the form of a panic attack.
   3. The person recognizes that the fear is excessive or unreasonable.
   4. The feared situations are avoided or endured with intense distress.
   5. The avoidance, anxious anticipation, or distress in the feared situations interferes with normal functioning or causes marked distress.
   6. The duration of symptoms is at least six months.
   7. The fear is not caused by a substance or medical condition and is not caused by another disorder.
   8. If a medical condition or another mental disorder is present, the fear is unrelated (eg, the fear is not of trembling in a patient with Parkinson's disease).
   9. Specify if the fear is generalized: The fear is generalized if the patient fears most social situations.

## II. Clinical Features of Social Phobia
   A. Patients often display hypersensitivity to criticism, difficulty being assertive, low self-esteem, and inadequate social skills.
   B. Avoidance of speaking in front of groups may lead to work or school difficulties. Most patients with social phobia fear public speaking, while less than half fear meeting new people.
   C. Less common fears include fear of eating, drinking, or writing in public, or of using a public restroom.

## III. Epidemiology and Etiology of Social Phobia
   A. Lifetime prevalence is 3-13%.
   B. Social phobia is more frequent (up to tenfold) in first-degree relatives of patients with generalized social phobia.
   C. Onset usually occurs in adolescence, with a childhood history of shyness.
   D. Social phobia is often a lifelong problem, but the disorder may remit or

improve in adulthood.
## IV. Differential Diagnosis of Social Phobia
    **A. Substance-Induced Anxiety Disorder.** Substances such as caffeine, amphetamines, cocaine, alcohol or benzodiazepines may cause a withdrawal syndrome that can mimic symptoms of social phobia

    **B. Obsessive-Compulsive Disorder, Specific Phobia, Hypochondriasis, or Anorexia Nervosa.** Anxiety symptoms are common in depression and the anxiety disorders. The diagnosis of social phobia should be made only if the anxiety is unrelated to another disorder. For example, social phobia should not be diagnosed in panic disorder if the patient has social restriction and excessive anxiety about having an attack in public.

    **C. Anxiety Disorder Due to a General Medical Condition.** Hyperthyroidism (and other medical conditions) may produce significant anxiety, and should be ruled out.

    **D. Mood and Psychotic Disorders.** Excessive social worry and anxiety can occur in many mood and psychotic disorders. If anxiety occurs only during the course of the mood or psychotic disorder, then social phobia should not be diagnosed.

## V. Treatment of Social Phobia
    **A.** SSRIs, such as paroxetine (Paxil) 20-40 mg/day or sertraline (Zoloft) 50-100 mg/day, are first-line medications for social phobia. Venlafaxine (Effexor XR) 75-225mg/day may also be used. Benzodiazepines, such as clonazepam (Klonopin) 0.5-2 mg per day, may be used if antidepressants are ineffective.

    **B.** Social phobia with performance anxiety (for specific situations known to be anxiety provoking) responds well to beta-blockers, such as propranolol. The effective dosage can be very low, such as 10-20 mg qid. It may also be used on a prn basis; 20-40 mg given 30-60 minutes prior to the anxiety provoking event.

    **C.** Cognitive/behavioral therapies are effective and should focus on cognitive retraining, desensitization, and relaxation techniques. Combined pharmacotherapy and cognitive or behavioral therapies is the most effective treatment.

# Specific Phobia

## I. DSM-IV Diagnostic Criteria
    **A.** Marked and persistent fear that is excessive or unreasonable, which is caused by the presence or anticipation of a specific object or situation.

    **B.** Exposure to the feared stimulus provokes an immediate anxiety response, which may take the form of a panic attack.

    **C.** Recognition by the patient that the fear is excessive or unreasonable.

    **D.** The phobic situation is avoided or endured with intense anxiety.

    **E.** The avoidance, anxious anticipation, or distress in the feared situations interferes with functioning or causes marked distress.

    **F.** In individuals under age 18, the duration must be at least six months.

    **G.** Symptoms are not caused by another mental disorder (eg, fear of dirt in someone with OCD).

    **H. Specify Types of Phobias**
        **1.** Animal (eg, dogs).
        **2.** Natural Environmental (eg, heights, storms, water).

   3. Blood-injection injury.
   4. Situational (eg, airplanes, elevators, enclosed places).
   5. Other (eg, situations that may lead to choking, vomiting).

## II. Clinical Features of Specific Phobia

   A. Specific phobias may result in a significant restriction of life-activities or occupation. Vasovagal fainting is seen in 75% of patients with blood-injection injury phobias.
   B. Specific phobias often occur along with other anxiety disorders.
   C. Many phobias do not come to clinical attention because they do not interfere with functioning.
   D. Fear of animals and other objects is common in childhood, and specific phobia is not diagnosed unless the fear leads to significant impairment, such as unwillingness to go to school.
   E. Most childhood phobias are self-limited and do not require treatment. Phobias that continue into adulthood rarely remit.

## III. Epidemiology of Specific Phobia

   A. The lifetime prevalence of phobias is 10%. Most do not cause clinically significant impairment or distress.
   B. Age of onset is variable, and females with the disorder far outnumber males.

## IV. Differential Diagnosis of Specific Phobia

   A. **Substance-Induced Anxiety Disorder.** Substances such as caffeine, amphetamines and cocaine can mimic phobic symptoms. Alcohol or benzodiazepine withdrawal can also mimic phobic symptoms.
   B. **Panic Disorder, Obsessive-Compulsive Disorder, Social Phobia, Hypochondriasis or Anorexia Nervosa.** Many psychiatric disorders present with marked anxiety, and the diagnosis of specific phobia should be made only if the anxiety is unrelated to another disorder. For example, phobias regarding eating or weight gain are not diagnosed if they are secondary to an underlying eating disorder.
   C. **Anxiety Disorder Due to a General Medical Condition.** Hyperthyroidism and other medical conditions may produce significant anxiety.
   D. **Mood and Psychotic Disorders.** Excessive worry and anxiety occurs in many mood and psychotic disorders. If anxiety occurs only during the course of the mood or psychotic disorder, then specific phobia should not be diagnosed.

## V. Treatment of Specific Phobia

   A. The primary treatment is behavioral therapy. A commonly used technique is systemic desensitization, consisting of gradually increasing exposure to the feared situation, combined with a relaxation technique such as deep breathing.
   B. Beta-blockers may also be useful prior to confronting the specific feared situation.

# Post-Traumatic Stress Disorder

## I. DSM-IV Diagnostic Criteria for Post-Traumatic Stress Disorder

   A. Post-traumatic stress disorder (PTSD) occurs after an individual has been exposed to a traumatic event that is associated with intense fear or horror.
   B. The patient persistently reexperiences the event through intrusive recollection or nightmares, reliving of the experience (flashbacks), or

intense distress when exposed to reminders of the event.

C. The patient may have feelings of detachment (emotional numbing), anhedonia, amnesia, restricted affect, or active avoidance of thoughts or activities that may be reminders of the trauma (three required).

D. A general state of increased arousal persists after the traumatic event, which is characterized by poor concentration, hypervigilance, exaggerated startle response, insomnia, or irritability (two required).

E. Symptoms have been present for at least one month.

F. Symptoms cause significant distress or impaired occupational or social functioning.

## II. Clinical Features of Post-Traumatic Stress Disorder

A. Survivor guilt (guilt over surviving when others have died) may be experienced if the trauma was associated with a loss of life.

B. Personality change, poor impulse control, aggression, dissociative symptoms, and perceptual disturbances may occur.

C. The risk of depression, substance abuse, other anxiety disorders, somatization disorder, and suicide are increased.

## III. Epidemiology of Post-Traumatic Stress Disorder

A. The lifetime prevalence of PTSD is 8% and is highest in young adults.

B. The prevalence in combat soldiers and assault victims is 60%.

C. Individuals with a personal history of maladaptive responses to stress may be predisposed to developing PTSD.

## IV. Classification of Post-Traumatic Stress Disorder

A. **Acute.** Symptoms have been present for less than three months.

B. **Chronic.** Symptoms have been present for greater than three months.

C. **With Delayed Onset.** Symptoms begin six months after the stressor.

## V. Differential Diagnosis of Post-Traumatic Stress Disorder

A. **Depression** is also associated with insomnia, anhedonia, poor concentration, and feelings of detachment. A stressful event may be associated with the onset of depression. Depression is not commonly associated with nightmares or flashbacks of a traumatic event.

B. **Obsessive-Compulsive Disorder.** OCD is associated with recurrent intrusive ideas. However, these ideas lack a relationship to a specific traumatic event, and the ideas are not usually recollections of past events.

C. **Malingering.** PTSD may be an illness for which monetary compensation is given. The presence of a primary financial gain for which patients may fabricate or exaggerate symptoms should be considered during evaluation.

D. **Anxiety Disorders.** Other anxiety disorders can cause symptoms of increased arousal, numbing, and avoidance. Symptoms, however, often were present before the traumatic event.

E. **Borderline Personality Disorder** can be associated with anhedonia, poor concentration, past history of emotional trauma and dissociative states similar to flashbacks. Other features of BPD such as avoidance of abandonment, identity disturbance, and impulsivity distinguishes BPD from PTSD.

## VI. Treatment of Post-Traumatic Stress Disorder

A. Sertraline (Zoloft) and paroxetine (Paxil) have demonstrated efficacy for all the symptom clusters of PTSD. Other SSRIs are also likely to be effective. Treatment at higher doses than are used for depression may be required. Older antidepressants (imipramine, amitriptyline, and monoamine oxidase inhibitors [MAOIs]) are moderately effective, especially for symptoms of increased arousal, intrusive thoughts, and coexisting

depression.
- **B.** Propranolol, lithium, anticonvulsants, and buspirone may be effective and should be considered if there is no response to antidepressants. Benzodiazepines are not effective for PTSD, except during the early, acute phase of the illness.
- **C.** Psychotherapy, behavioral therapy, support groups, and family therapy are effective adjuncts to pharmacological treatment.

# Acute Stress Disorder

Acute stress disorder may occur as an acute reaction following exposure to extreme stress.

**I. DSM-IV Criteria for Acute Stress Disorder.**
- **A.** Symptoms described below occur after an individual has been exposed to a traumatic event that is outside the realm of normal human experience (combat, natural disaster, physical assault, accident).
- **B.** The patient persistently reexperiences the event through intrusive recollection or nightmares, reliving of the experience (flashbacks), or intense distress when exposed to reminders of the event.
- **C.** Persistent avoidance of the traumatic event and emotional numbing (feeling of detachment from others) may be present. The patient may have feelings of detachment, anhedonia, amnesia, restricted affect, or active avoidance of thoughts or activities that may be reminders of the trauma (three required).
- **D.** A general state of increased arousal persists after the traumatic event, which is characterized by poor concentration, hypervigilance, exaggerated startle response, insomnia or irritability (two required).
- **E.** Additional findings in acute stress disorder may include the following:
  - **1.** Symptoms occur within one month of a stressor and last between two days and four weeks.
  - **2.** The individual has three or more of the following dissociative symptoms:
    - **a.** Subjective sense of numbing, detachment or absence of emotional responsiveness.
    - **b.** Reduction in awareness of surroundings.
    - **c.** Derealization.
    - **d.** Depersonalization.
    - **e.** Dissociative amnesia.

**II. Treatment of Acute Stress Disorder**
- **A.** The presence of acute stress disorder may precede PTSD. The clinical approach to acute stress disorder is similar to PTSD.
- **B.** Treatment of acute stress disorder consists of supportive psychotherapy.
- **C.** Sedative hypnotics are indicated for short-term treatment of insomnia and symptoms of increased arousal. Antidepressant medications are indicated if these agents are ineffective.

### References
References, see page 120.

# *Personality Disorders*

---

I. **General Characteristics of Personality Disorders**
   A. Personality traits consist of enduring patterns of perceiving, relating to, and thinking about the environment, other people and oneself.
   B. A personality disorder is diagnosed when personality traits become inflexible, pervasive and maladaptive to the point where they cause significant social or occupational dysfunction or subjective distress. Patients usually have little or no insight into their disorder.
   C. Personality patterns must be stable and date back to adolescence or early adulthood. Therefore, personality disorders are not generally diagnosed in children.
   D. Patterns of behavior and perception cannot be caused by stress, another mental disorder, drug or medication effect, or a medical condition.

## Cluster A Personality Disorders

Paranoid, schizotypal and schizoid personality disorders are referred to as cluster A personality disorders. Patients with these disorders have a preference for social isolation. There is also an increased incidence of schizophrenia in first-degree relatives compared to the general population. Patients with cluster A personality disorders often develop schizophrenia. They are considered part of the schizophrenia-spectrum disorders, possibly milder variants of schizophrenia.

## Paranoid Personality Disorder

I. **DSM-IV Diagnostic Criteria of Paranoid Personality Disorder**
   A. A pervasive distrust and suspiciousness of others is present without justification, beginning by early adulthood, and is manifested by at least four of the following:
      1. The patient suspects others are exploiting, harming, or deceiving him.
      2. The patient doubts the loyalty or trustworthiness of others.
      3. The patient fears that information given to others will be used maliciously against him.
      4. Benign remarks by others or benign events are interpreted as having demeaning or threatening meanings.
      5. The patient persistently bears grudges.
      6. The patient perceives attacks that are not apparent to others, and is quick to react angrily or to counterattack.
      7. The patient repeatedly questions the fidelity of his spouse or sexual partner.
II. **Clinical Features of Paranoid Personality Disorder**
   A. The patient is often hypervigilant and constantly looking for proof to support his paranoia. Patients are often argumentative and hostile.
   B. Patients have a high need for control and autonomy in relationships to avoid betrayal and the need to trust others. Pathological jealousy is common.

C. Patients are quick to counterattack and are frequently involved in legal disputes. These patients rarely seek treatment.

### III. Epidemiology of Paranoid Personality Disorder
   A. The disorder is more common in first-degree relatives of schizophrenics compared to the general population.
   B. Patients with the disorder may develop schizophrenia.
   C. The disorder is more common in men than women.

### IV. Differential Diagnosis of Paranoid Personality Disorder
   A. **Delusional Disorder.** Fixed delusions are not seen in personality disorders.
   B. **Paranoid Schizophrenia.** Hallucinations and formal thought disorder are not seen in personality disorder.
   C. **Personality Change Due to a General Medical Condition and Substance-Related Disorder.** Acute symptoms are temporally related to a medication, drugs or a medical condition. The longstanding patterns of behavior required for a personality disorder are not present.

### V. Treatment of Paranoid Personality Disorder
   A. Psychotherapy is the treatment of choice for PPD, but establishing and maintaining the trust of patients may be difficult because these patients have great difficulty tolerating intimacy.
   B. Symptoms of anxiety and agitation may be severe enough to warrant treatment with antianxiety agents.
   C. Low doses of antipsychotics are useful for delusional accusations and agitation.

# Schizoid Personality Disorder

### I. DSM-IV Diagnostic Criteria for Schizoid Personality Disorder
   A. A pervasive pattern of social detachment with restricted affect, beginning by early adulthood and indicated by at least four of the following:
      1. The patient neither desires nor enjoys close relationships, including family relationships.
      2. The patient chooses solitary activities.
      3. The patient has little interest in having sexual experiences.
      4. The patient takes pleasure in few activities.
      5. The patient has no close friends or confidants except first-degree relatives.
      6. The patient is indifferent to the praise or criticism of others.
      7. The patient displays emotional detachment or diminished affective responsiveness.

### II. Clinical Features of Schizoid Personality Disorder
   A. The patient often appears cold and aloof, and is uninvolved in the everyday concerns of others.
   B. Patients with SPD are often emotionally blunted, and these patients generally do not marry unless pursued aggressively by another person.
   C. These patients are able to work if the job allows for social isolation.

### III. Epidemiology of Schizoid Personality Disorder
   A. Schizoid Personality Disorder is more common in first-degree relatives of schizophrenics compared to the general public.
   B. Patients with Schizoid Personality Disorder may develop schizophrenia.
   C. Schizoid Personality Disorder is a rare disorder, which is thought to be

more common in men than women.

## IV. Differential Diagnosis of Schizoid Personality Disorder

A. **Schizophrenia.** Hallucinations and formal thought disorder are not seen in personality disorders. Patients with schizoid personality disorder may have good work histories, whereas schizophrenic patients usually have poor work histories.

B. **Schizotypal Personality Disorder.** Eccentricities and oddities of perception, behavior and speech are not seen in schizoid personality disorder.

C. **Avoidant Personality Disorder.** Social isolation is subjectively unpleasant for avoidant patients. Unlike schizoid patients, avoidant patients are hypersensitive to the thoughts and feelings of others.

D. **Paranoid Personality Disorder.** Paranoid patients are able to express strong emotion when they feel persecuted. Schizoid patients are not able to express strong emotion.

E. **Personality Change Due to a General Medical Condition and Substance-Related Disorder.** Acute symptoms are temporally related to a medication, drugs or a medical condition. The longstanding patterns of behavior required for a personality disorder are not present.

## V. Treatment of Schizoid Personality Disorder

A. Individual psychotherapy is the treatment of choice. Group therapy is not recommended because other patients will find the patient's silence difficult to tolerate.

B. The use of antidepressants, antipsychotics and psychostimulants has been described without consistent results.

# Schizotypal Personality Disorder

## I. DSM-IV Diagnostic Criteria

A. A pervasive pattern of discomfort with and reduced capacity for close relationships as well as perceptual distortions and eccentricities of behavior, beginning by early adulthood. At least five of the following should be present:

1. **Ideas of reference:** interpreting unrelated events as having direct reference to the patient (eg, belief that a television program is really about him).

2. Odd beliefs or magical thinking inconsistent with cultural norms (eg, superstitiousness, belief in clairvoyance, telepathy or a "sixth sense").

3. Unusual perceptual experiences, including bodily illusions.

4. Odd thinking and speech (eg, circumstantial, metaphorical or stereotyped thinking).

5. Suspiciousness or paranoid ideation.

6. Inappropriate or constricted affect.

7. Behavior or appearance that is odd, eccentric or peculiar.

8. Lack of close friends other than first-degree relatives.

9. Excessive social anxiety that does not diminish with familiarity.

## II. Clinical Features of Schizotypal Personality Disorder

A. These patients often display peculiarities in thinking, behavior and communication.

B. Discomfort in social situations, and inappropriate behavior may occur.

C. Magical thinking, belief in "extra sensory perception," illusions and

      derealization are common.
- **D.** Repeated exposure will not decrease social anxiety since it is based on paranoid concerns and not on self-consciousness.
- **E.** The patient may have a vivid fantasy life with imaginary relationships.
- **F.** Speech may be idiosyncratic, such as the use of unusual terminology.
- **G.** These patients may seek treatment for anxiety or depression.

### III. Epidemiology of Schizotypal Personality Disorder
- **A.** This disorder is more common in first-degree relatives of schizophrenics compared to the general population.
- **B.** Patients with schizotypal personality disorder may develop schizophrenia.
- **C.** The prevalence is approximately 3% in the general population.  ·

### IV. Differential Diagnosis of Schizotypal Personality Disorder
- **A. Schizoid and Avoidant Personality Disorder.** Schizoid and avoidant patients will not display the oddities of behavior, perception, and communication of schizotypal patients.
- **B. Schizophrenia.** No formal thought disorder is present in personality disorders. When psychosis is present in schizotypal patients, it is of brief duration.
- **C. Paranoid Personality Disorder.** Patients with paranoid personality disorder will not display the oddities of behavior, perception and communication of schizotypal patients. Unlike schizotypals, paranoid patients can be very verbally aggressive and do not avoid conflict.
- **D. Personality Change Due to a General Medical Condition and Substance-Related Disorder.** Acute symptoms are temporally related to a medication, drugs or a medical condition. The longstanding patterns of behavior required for a personality disorder are not present.

### V. Treatment of Schizotypal Personality Disorder
- **A.** Psychotherapy is the treatment of choice for schizotypal personality disorder. Antipsychotics may be helpful in dealing with low-grade psychotic symptoms or paranoid delusions.
- **B.** Antidepressants may be useful if the patient also meets criteria for a mood disorder.

# Cluster B Personality Disorders

Antisocial, borderline, histrionic and narcissistic personality disorders are referred to as cluster B personality disorders. These disorders are characterized by dramatic or irrational behavior. These patients tend to be very disruptive in clinical settings.

# Antisocial Personality Disorder

I. **DSM-IV Diagnostic Criteria for Antisocial Personality Disorder**
  A. Since age 15 years, the patient has exhibited disregard for and violation of the rights of others, indicated by at least three of the following:
    1. Failure to conform to social norms by repeatedly engaging in unlawful activity.
    2. Deceitfulness: repeated lying or "conning" others for profit or pleasure.
    3. Impulsivity or failure to plan ahead.
    4. Irritability and aggressiveness, such as repeated physical fighting or assaults.
    5. Reckless disregard for the safety of self or others.
    6. Consistent irresponsibility: repeated failure to sustain consistent work or honor financial obligations.
    7. Lack of remorse for any of the above behavior.
  B. A history of some symptoms of conduct disorder before age 15 years as indicated by:
    1. Aggression to people and animals.
    2. Destruction of property.
    3. Deceitfulness or theft.
    4. Serious violation of rules.
II. **Clinical Features of Antisocial Personality Disorder**
  A. Interactions with others are typically exploitative or abusive.
  B. Lying, stealing, fighting, fraud, physical abuse, substance abuse, and drunk driving are common.
  C. Patients may be arrogant, but they are also capable of great superficial charm.
  D. These patients do not have a capacity for empathy.
III. **Epidemiology of Antisocial Personality Disorder**
  A. The male-to-female ratio is 3:1.
  B. APD is more common in first-degree relatives of those with the disorder.
IV. **Differential Diagnosis of Antisocial Personality Disorder**
  A. **Adult Antisocial Behavior.** This diagnosis is limited to the presence of illegal behavior only. Patients with adult antisocial behavior do not show the pervasive, long-term patterns required for a personality disorder.
  B. **Substance-Related Disorder.** Substance abuse is common in antisocial personality disorder, and crimes may be committed to obtain drugs or to obtain money for drugs. Many patients will meet criteria for both diagnoses.
  C. **Narcissistic Personality Disorder.** Narcissistic patients also lack empathy and are exploitative, but they are not as aggressive or deceitful as antisocial patients.
  D. **Borderline Personality Disorder.** These patients are also impulsive and

manipulative, but they are more emotionally unstable and they are less aggressive. The manipulativeness of borderline patients is aimed at getting emotional gratification rather than aimed at financial motivations.

## V. Treatment of Antisocial Personality Disorder
- A. These patients will try to destroy or avoid the therapeutic relationship. Inpatient self-help groups are the most useful treatment because the patient is not allowed to leave, and because enhanced peer interaction minimizes authority issues.
- B. Psychotropic medication is used in patients whose symptoms interfere with functioning or who meet criteria for another psychiatric disorder. Anticonvulsants, lithium, and beta-blockers have been used for impulse control problems, including rage reactions. Antidepressants can be helpful if depression or an anxiety disorder is present.

# Borderline Personality Disorder

## I. DSM-IV Diagnostic Criteria for Borderline Personality Disorder
A pervasive pattern of unstable interpersonal relationships, unstable self-image, unstable affects, and poor impulse control, beginning by early adulthood, and indicated by at least five of the following:
1. Frantic efforts to avoid real or imagined abandonment.
2. Unstable and intense interpersonal relationships, alternating between extremes of idealization and devaluation.
3. Identity disturbance: unstable self-image or sense of self.
4. Impulsivity in at least two areas that are potentially self-damaging (eg, spending, promiscuity, substance abuse, reckless driving, binge eating).
5. Recurrent suicidal behavior, gestures or threats; or self-mutilating behavior.
6. Affective instability (eg, sudden intense dysphoria, irritability or anxiety of short duration).
7. Chronic feelings of emptiness.
8. Inappropriate, intense anger or difficulty controlling anger.
9. Transient, stress-related paranoid ideation, or severe dissociative symptoms.

## II. Clinical Features of Borderline Personality Disorder
- A. The clinical presentation of BPD is highly variable. Chronic dysphoria is common, and desperate dependence on others is caused by inability to tolerate being alone.
- B. Chaotic interpersonal relationships are characteristic, and self-destructive or self-mutilatory behavior is common.
- C. A childhood history of abuse or parental neglect is common.

## III. Epidemiology of Borderline Personality Disorder
- A. The female-to-male ratio is 2:1. The disorder is five times more common in first-degree relatives.
- B. The prevalence is 1-2%, but the disorder occurs in 30-60% of psychiatric patients.

IV. **Differential Diagnosis of Borderline Personality Disorder**
  A. **Adolescence.** Normal adolescence with identity disturbance and emotional lability shares many of the same characteristics of BPD; however, the longstanding pervasive pattern of behavior required for a personality disorder is not present.
  B. **Histrionic Personality Disorder.** These patients are also manipulative and attention seeking, but they do not display self-destructiveness and rage. Psychosis and dissociation are not typically seen in histrionic patients.
  C. **Dependent Personality Disorder.** When faced with abandonment, dependent patients will increase their submissive behavior rather than display rage as do borderline patients.
  D. **Personality Change Due to a General Medical Condition and Substance-Related Disorder.** Acute symptoms are temporally related to medications, drugs, or a medical condition.
V. **Treatment of Borderline Personality Disorder**
  A. Psychotherapy is the treatment of choice. Patients frequently try to recreate their personal chaos in treatment by displaying acting-out behavior, resistance to treatment, lability of mood and affect, and regression.
  B. Suicide threats and attempts are common.
  C. Pharmacotherapy is frequently used for coexisting mood disorders, eating disorders, and anxiety disorders. Valproate (Depakote) or SSRIs may be helpful for impulsive-aggressive behavior.

# Histrionic Personality Disorder

I. **DSM-IV Diagnostic Criteria**
  A. A pervasive pattern of excessive emotionality and attention seeking, beginning by early adulthood, as indicated by five or more of the following:
     1. The patient is not comfortable unless he is the center of attention.
     2. The patient is often inappropriately sexually seductive or provocative with others.
     3. Rapidly shifting and shallow expression of emotions are present.
     4. The patient consistently uses physical appearance to attract attention.
     5. Speech is excessively impressionistic and lacking in detail.
     6. Dramatic, theatrical, and exaggerated expression of emotion is used.
     7. The patient is easily influenced by others or by circumstances.
     8. Relationships are considered to be more intimate than they are in reality.
II. **Clinical Features of Histrionic Personality Disorder**
  A. The patient is bored with routine and dislikes delays in gratification.
  B. The patient begins projects, but does not finish them (including relationships).
  C. Dramatic emotional "performances" of the patient appear to lack sincerity.
  D. These patients often attempt to control relationships with seduction, manipulation, or dependency.
  E. The patient may resort to suicidal gestures and threats to get attention.

### III. Epidemiology of Histrionic Personality Disorder
    **A.** The prevalence of HPD is 2-3%.
    **B.** Histrionic personality disorder is much more common in women than men.
    **C.** These patients have higher rates of depression, somatization and conversion disorder compared to the general population.

### IV. Differential Diagnosis of Histrionic Personality Disorder
    **A. Borderline Personality Disorder**
      **1.** While patients with Borderline Personality can also be sensation-seeking, impulsive, superficially charming, and manipulative, they also have identity disturbance, transient psychosis, and dissociation, which are not seen in histrionic patients.
      **2.** Some patients meet criteria for both BPD and HPD.
    **B. Antisocial Personality Disorder**
      **1.** Antisocial patients are also sensation-seeking, impulsive, superficially charming, and manipulative.
      **2.** Histrionic patients are dramatic and theatrical but typically lack histories of antisocial behavior.
    **C. Narcissistic Personality Disorder**
      **1.** Narcissists also seek constant attention, but it must be positive in order to confirm grandiosity and superiority.
      **2.** Histrionics are less selective and will readily appear weak and dependent in order to get attention.
    **D. Personality Change Due to a General Medical Condition and Substance-Related Disorder.** Acute symptoms are temporally related to medication, drugs, or a medical condition.

### V. Treatment of Histrionic Personality Disorder
    **A.** Insight-oriented psychotherapy is the treatment of choice. Keeping patients in therapy can be challenging since these patients dislike routine.
    **B.** Antidepressants are used if depression is also present.

# Narcissistic Personality Disorder

### I. DSM-IV Diagnostic Criteria
    **A.** A pervasive pattern of grandiosity (in fantasy or behavior), need for admiration, and lack of empathy. The disorder begins by early adulthood and is indicated by at least five of the following:
      **1.** An exaggerated sense of self-importance.
      **2.** Preoccupation with fantasies of unlimited success, power, brilliance, beauty, or ideal love.
      **3.** Believes he is "special" and can only be understood by, or should associate with, other special or high-status people (or institutions).
      **4.** Requires excessive admiration.
      **5.** Has a sense of entitlement.
      **6.** Takes advantage of others to achieve his own ends.
      **7.** Lacks empathy.
      **8.** The patient is often envious of others or believes that others are envious of him.
      **9.** Shows arrogant, haughty behavior or attitudes.

II. **Clinical Features of Narcissistic Personality Disorder**
   A. Patients with narcissistic personality disorder exaggerate their achievements and talents, and they are surprised when they do not receive the recognition they expect.
   B. Their inflated sense of self results in a devaluation of others and their accomplishments. Narcissistic patients only pursue relationships that will benefit them in some way.
   C. These patients feel very entitled, expecting others to meet their needs immediately, and they can become quite indignant if this does not happen. These patients are self-absorbed and unable to respond to the needs of others. Any perception of criticism is poorly tolerated, and these patients can react with rage.
   D. These patients are very prone to envy anyone who possesses knowledge, skill or belongings that they do not possess. Much of narcissistic behavior serves as a defense against very poor self-esteem.

III. **Epidemiology of Narcissistic Personality Disorder**
   A. The prevalence of NPD is less than 1% in the general population and up to 16% in clinical populations.
   B. The disorder is more common in men than women. Studies have shown a steady increase in the incidence of narcissistic personality disorder.

IV. **Differential Diagnosis of Narcissistic Personality Disorder**
   A. **Histrionic Personality Disorder.** Histrionic patients are also attention seeking, but the attention they seek does not need to be admiring. They are more highly emotional and seductive compared to patients with NPD.
   B. **Borderline Personality Disorder.** These patients also tend to idealize and devalue others, but narcissistic patients lack the unstable identity, self-destructive behavior, and abandonment fears that characterize borderline patients.
   C. **Antisocial Personality Disorder.** Interpersonal exploitation, superficial charm, and lack of empathy can be seen in both antisocial personality disorder and narcissistic personality disorder. However, antisocial patients do not require constant admiration nor do they display the envy seen in narcissistic patients.
   D. **Personality Change Due to a General Medical Condition and Substance-Related Disorder.** All symptoms are temporally related to medication, drugs or a medical condition.

V. **Treatment of Narcissistic Personality Disorder**
   A. Psychotherapy is the treatment of choice, but the therapeutic relationship can be difficult since envy often becomes an issue.
   B. Coexisting substance abuse may complicate treatment. Depression frequently coexists with NPD; therefore, antidepressants are useful for adjunctive therapy.

# Cluster C Personality Disorders

Avoidant, dependent and obsessive-compulsive personality disorders are referred to as cluster C personality disorders. These patients tend to be anxious and their personality pathology is a maladaptive attempt to control anxiety.

# Avoidant Personality Disorder

I. **DSM-IV Diagnostic Criteria**
    A. A pervasive pattern of social inhibition, feelings of inadequacy and hypersensitivity, beginning by early adulthood, and indicated by at least four of the following:
        1. The patient avoids occupational activities with significant interpersonal contact due to fear of criticism, disapproval or rejection.
        2. Unwilling to get involved with people unless certain of being liked.
        3. Restrained in intimate relationships due to fear of being shamed or ridiculed.
        4. Preoccupied with being criticized or rejected in social situations.
        5. Inhibited in new interpersonal situations due to feelings of inadequacy.
        6. The patient views himself as socially inept, unappealing or inferior to others.
        7. Reluctance to take personal risks or to engage in new activities because they may be embarrassing.
II. **Clinical Features of Avoidant Personality Disorder**
    A. The patient is usually shy and quiet and prefers to be alone. The patient usually anticipates unwarranted rejection before it happens.
    B. Opportunities to supervise others at work are usually avoided by the patient. These patients are often devastated by minor comments they perceive to be critical.
    C. Despite self-imposed restrictions, avoidant personality disorder patients usually long to be accepted and be more social.
III. **Epidemiology of Avoidant Personality Disorder**
    A. The male-to-female ratio is 1:1.
    B. Although adults with avoidant personality disorder were frequently shy as children, childhood shyness is not a predisposing factor.
IV. **Differential Diagnosis of Avoidant Personality Disorder**
    A. **Social Phobia, Generalized Type** shares many features of avoidant personality disorder. Patients may meet criteria for both disorders. The two disorders may only be differentiated by a life-long pattern of avoidance seen in patients with avoidant personality disorder.
    B. **Dependent Personality Disorder.** These patients are also hypersensitive to criticism and crave acceptance, but they will risk humiliation and rejection in order to get their dependent needs met. Patients may meet the criteria for both disorders.
    C. **Schizoid Personality Disorder**. These patients also avoid interactions with others and are anxious in social settings; however, schizoid patients do not fear criticism and rejection. Avoidant patients recognize that social isolation is abnormal.
    D. **Panic Disorder with Agoraphobia.** In patients with panic disorder with agoraphobia, avoidance occurs after the panic attack has begun, and the

avoidance is aimed at preventing another panic attack from occurring.
## V. Treatment of Avoidant Personality Disorder
  A. Individual psychotherapy, group psychotherapy and behavioral techniques may all be useful. Group therapy may assist in dealing with social anxiety. Behavioral techniques, such as assertiveness training and systematic desensitization, may help the patient to overcome anxiety and shyness.
  B. Beta-blockers can be useful for situational anxiety.
  C. Since many of these patients will meet criteria for Social Phobia (generalized), a trial of SSRI medication may prove beneficial. Patients are prone to other mood and anxiety disorders, and these disorders should be treated with antidepressants or anxiolytics.

# Dependent Personality Disorder

## I. DSM-IV Diagnostic Criteria
  A. A pervasive and excessive need to be cared for. This need leads to submissive, clinging behavior, and fears of separation beginning by early adulthood and indicated by at least five of the following:
    1. Difficulty making everyday decisions without excessive advice and reassurance.
    2. Needs others to assume responsibility for major areas of his life.
    3. Difficulty expressing disagreement with others and unrealistically fears loss of support or approval if he disagrees.
    4. Difficulty initiating projects or doing things on his or her own because of a lack of self-confidence in judgment or abilities.
    5. Goes to excessive lengths to obtain nurturance and support, to the point of volunteering to do things that are unpleasant.
    6. Uncomfortable or helpless when alone due to exaggerated fears of being unable to care for himself.
    7. Urgently seeks another source of care and support when a close relationship ends.
    8. Unrealistically preoccupied with fears of being left to take care of himself.

## II. Clinical Features of Dependent Personality Disorder
  A. Patients will endure great discomfort in order to perpetuate the care-taking relationship. Social interaction is usually limited to the caretaker network.
  B. These patients may function at work if no initiative is required.

## III. Epidemiology of Dependent Personality Disorder
  A. Women are affected slightly more than men.
  B. Childhood illness or separation anxiety disorder of childhood predispose patients to dependent personality disorder.

## IV. Differential Diagnosis of Dependent Personality Disorder
  A. **Avoidant Personality Disorder.** Avoidant patients are more focused on avoiding shame and rejection rather than getting needs met. Some patients may meet criteria for both disorders.
  B. **Borderline Personality Disorder.** Borderline patients react with rage and emptiness when feeling abandoned. Dependent patients react with more submissive behavior when feeling abandoned.
  C. **Histrionic Personality Disorder.** These patients are also needy and

clinging, and they have a strong desire for approval, but these patients actively pursue almost any kind of attention. They tend to be very flamboyant, unlike dependent patients.

    **D. Personality Change Due to a General Medical Condition and Substance-Related Disorder.** Acute symptoms are temporally related to a medication, drugs or a medical condition.

**V. Treatment of Dependent Personality Disorder**

    **A.** Insight-oriented psychotherapy, group, and behavioral therapies, such as assertiveness and social skills training, have all been used with success. Family therapy may also be helpful in supporting new needs of the dependent patient in treatment.

    **B.** Dependent patients are at increased risk for mood disorders and anxiety disorders. Appropriate pharmacological interventions may be used if the patient has these disorders.

# Obsessive-Compulsive Personality Disorder

**I. DSM-IV Diagnostic Criteria**

    **A.** A pervasive pattern of preoccupation with orderliness, perfectionism and control, at the expense of flexibility, openness, and efficiency, beginning by early adulthood and indicated by at least four of the following:

        **1.** Preoccupied with details, rules, lists, organization or schedules, to the extent that the major point of the activity is lost.

        **2.** Perfectionism interferes with task completion.

        **3.** Excessively devoted to work and productivity to the exclusion of leisure activities and friendships.

        **4.** Overconscientiousness, scrupulousness and inflexibility about morality, ethics, or values (not accounted for by culture or religion).

        **5.** Unable to discard worn-out or worthless objects, even if they have no sentimental value.

        **6.** Reluctant to delegate tasks to others.

        **7.** Miserly spending style toward both self and others.

        **8.** Rigidity and stubbornness.

**II. Clinical Features of Obsessive-Compulsive Personality Disorder (OCPD)**

    **A.** Obsession with detail can paralyze decision making.

    **B.** Tasks may be difficult to complete. These patients prefer logic and intellect to feelings, and they are not able to be openly affectionate.

    **C.** These patients are often very "frugal" with regard to financial matters.

**III. Epidemiology of Obsessive-Compulsive Personality Disorder**

    **A.** The prevalence of OCPD is 1% in the general population and up to 10% in clinical populations.

    **B.** The male-to-female ratio is 2:1.

    **C.** Obsessive-compulsive personality disorder is more frequent in first-degree relatives.

**IV. Differential Diagnosis of Obsessive-Compulsive Personality Disorder**

    **A. Obsessive-Compulsive Disorder (OCD).** Most patients with OCD do not meet criteria for OCPD, although the two conditions can coexist.

    **B. Personality Change Due to a General Medical Condition and Substance-Related Disorder.** Acute symptoms are temporally related to a medication, drugs, or a medical condition. The longstanding patterns of behavior required for a personality disorder are not present.

V. **Treatment of Obsessive-Compulsive Personality Disorder.** Long-term, individual therapy is usually helpful. Therapy can be difficult due to the patient's limited insight and rigidity.

### References
References, see page 120.

# *Somatoform and Factitious Disorders*

## Somatization Disorder

I. **DSM-IV Criteria**
   A. Many physical complaints, resulting in treatment being sought or significant functional impairment. Onset is before the age of 30.
   B. **Physical Complaints**
      1. History of pain related to at least four sites or functions.
      2. Two GI symptoms.
      3. One sexual symptom.
      4. One symptom suggestive of a neurological condition (pseudo-neurological).
   C. Symptoms cannot be explained by organic etiology or symptoms are in excess of what is expected from the medical evaluation.
   D. Symptoms are not intentionally produced.

II. **Clinical Features of Somatization Disorder**
   A. Somatization disorder is a chronic problem, and patients frequently seek medical treatment or pursue multiple concurrent treatments. Patients undergo multiple procedures, surgeries, and hospitalizations. The disorder often begins during adolescence.
   B. Frequently encountered symptoms include nausea, vomiting, extremity pain, shortness of breath, and pregnancy or menstruation associated complaints.
   C. The frequency and severity of symptoms may vary with level of stress.
   D. Two-thirds of patients have coexisting psychiatric diagnoses. Mood and anxiety disorders and substance-related disorders are common in somatization disorder.

III. **Epidemiology of Somatization Disorder**
   A. The lifetime prevalence is 0.1 to 0.5%. The disorder is 5-20 times more prevalent in women. The frequency of Somatization Disorder is inversely related to social class.
   B. Fifteen percent of patients have a positive family history, and the concordance rate is higher in monozygotic twins.

IV. **Differential Diagnosis of Somatization Disorder**
   A. Medical conditions that present varied symptoms, such as systemic lupus erythematosus, HIV or multiple sclerosis, must be excluded.
   B. Prominent somatic complaints can also be associated with depression, anxiety, and schizophrenia.
   C. **Malingering** is suspected when there are external motives (eg, financial) that would be furthered by the intentional production of symptoms.
   D. **Factitious Disorder**. In factitious disorder symptoms are intentionally produced to assume the sick role to meet a psychological need.

V. **Treatment of Somatization Disorder**
   A. The physical complaints that occur in somatization disorder are an expression of emotional issues. Psychotherapy is beneficial to help the patient find more appropriate and direct ways of expressing their emotional needs. Behaviorally oriented group therapy is also helpful.

**B.** The patient should have a primary care physician and should be seen at regular intervals to minimize inappropriate use of medical services.

# Conversion Disorder

## I. DSM-IV Criteria for Conversion Disorder
**A.** The patient complains of symptoms or deficits affecting voluntary muscles, or deficits of sensory function that suggest a neurological or medical condition.
**B.** The temporal relation of symptoms to a stressful event suggests association of psychological factors.
**C.** Symptoms are not intentionally produced.
**D.** Symptoms are not explained by an organic etiology.
**E.** Symptoms result in significant functional impairment.
**F.** Symptoms are not limited to pain or sexual dysfunction, and are not explained by another mental disorder.

## II. Clinical Features of Conversion Disorder
**A.** The most common symptoms are sensory (blindness, numbness) and motor deficits (paralysis, mutism), and pseudoseizures. Other symptoms include pseudocyesis (pregnancy), urinary retention, torticollis and voluntary motor paralysis (astasia-abasia).
**B.** Abnormalities usually do not have a normal anatomical distribution and the neurological exam is normal. Deficits tend to change over time.
**C.** Patients often lack the characteristic normal concern about the deficit. This characteristic lack of concern has been termed "la belle indifference." Conversion disorder can coexist with depression, anxiety disorders, and schizophrenia.
**D.** Conversion symptoms often will temporarily remit after the disorder has been suggested by the physician.

## III. Epidemiology of Conversion Disorder
**A.** Conversion disorder occurs in 1-30/10,000 in the general population and in up to 3% of outpatient psychiatric patients.
**B.** The disorder is more common in lower socioeconomic groups.

## IV. Differential Diagnosis of Conversion Disorder
**A. Medical conditions** must be excluded.
**B. Somatization Disorder** begins in early life and involves multi-organ symptoms. Patients tend to be very concerned about symptoms.
**C. Factitious Disorder.** Symptoms are under conscious voluntary control, and they are intentionally created to assume a sick role. In conversion disorder, symptoms are not consciously produced.
**D. Malingering** is characterized by the presence of external motivations behind fabrication of symptoms.

## V. Treatment of Conversion Disorder
**A.** Symptoms typically last for days to weeks and typically remit spontaneously. Supportive, insight-oriented or behavioral therapy can facilitate recovery.
**B.** Anxiolytics and relaxation may also be helpful in some cases. The physician should avoid confrontation or focusing on the symptoms. The focus should be on psychological issues and any secondary gain. Benzodiazepines can be useful when anxiety symptoms are prominent.

# Hypochondriasis

## I. DSM-IV Criteria for Hypochondriasis
   **A.** Preoccupation with fear of having a serious disease, based on misinterpretation of symptoms.
   **B.** The patient is not reassured by a negative medical evaluation.
   **C.** Symptoms are not related to delusions or restricted to specific concern about appearance.
   **D.** The disorder results in significant functional impairment.
   **E.** Duration is greater than six months.
   **F.** Symptoms are not accounted for by another mental disorder.

## II. Clinical Features of Hypochondriasis
   **A.** Despite clinical, diagnostic or laboratory evaluation, the patient is not reassured. Doctor shopping is common, and complaints are often vague and ambiguous.
   **B.** Repeated diagnostic procedures may result in unrelated medical complications.

## III. Epidemiology and Classification of Hypochondriasis
   **A.** The prevalence ranges from 4-9%. Hypochondriasis is most frequent between age 20 to 30 years, and there is no sex predominance.
   **B.** Hypochondriasis "with poor insight" is present if the patient fails to recognize that his concern about health is excessive or unreasonable.

## IV. Differential Diagnosis of Hypochondriasis
   **A.** Major depression, obsessive-compulsive disorder, generalized anxiety disorder, and panic disorder can often cause prominent somatic complaints with no organic basis.
   **B.** **Medical conditions** that can produce varied symptoms, such as AIDS, multiple sclerosis, and systemic lupus erythematosus, must be excluded.
   **C.** **Body Dysmorphic Disorder.** Concerns are limited only to physical appearance, in contrast to the fear of having an illness that occurs in hypochondriasis.
   **D.** **Factitious Disorder and Malingering.** Hypochondriacal patients realistically experience the symptoms and do not fabricate them.
   **E.** **Conversion Disorder.** This disorder tends to cause only one symptom, and the patient has less concern about the symptom.
   **F.** **Somatization Disorder.** The focus of the patient is on the symptoms, as opposed to fear of having a disease in hypochondriasis.

## V. Treatment of Hypochondriasis
   **A.** Improvement usually results from reassurance through regular physician visits. Cognitive-behavioral group therapy, rather than individual therapy, is most helpful.
   **B.** Coexisting psychiatric conditions should be treated. Hypochondriasis is sometimes episodic, and it may be related to stressful life events. There is preliminary evidence that SSRI medications are beneficial.

# Body Dysmorphic Disorder

I. **DSM-IV Criteria for Body Dysmorphic Disorder**
   A. A preoccupation with imagined defect in appearance.
   B. The preoccupation causes significant functional impairment.
   C. Preoccupation is not caused for by another mental disorder.

II. **Clinical Features of Body Dysmorphic Disorder**
   A. Facial features, hair, and body build are the most frequently "defective" features. Concerns about the imagined defect may reach delusional proportions without meeting criteria for a psychotic disorder. Multiple visits to surgeons and dermatologists are common.
   B. Major depressive disorder and anxiety disorders frequently coexist with body dysmorphic disorder.

III. **Epidemiology of Body Dysmorphic Disorder**
   A. The disorder is most common between the ages of 15 and 20 years, with women affected as frequently as men.
   B. Family history reflects a higher incidence of mood disorders and obsessive-compulsive disorder (OCD).

IV. **Differential Diagnosis of Body Dysmorphic Disorder**
   A. Neurological "neglect" is seen in parietal lobe lesions, and it can be mistaken for dysmorphic disorder.
   B. **Anorexia Nervosa.** Preoccupation about body image are limited to concerns about being "fat."
   C. **Gender Identity Disorder.** Characterized by discomfort with the patient's own sex and persistent identification with the opposite sex.
   D. **Narcissistic Personality Disorder.** In this disorder, concern with a body part is only one feature in broad constellation of other personality features.

V. **Treatment of Body Dysmorphic Disorder.** SSRI antidepressants and clomipramine are effective in reducing symptoms in 50% of patients, possibly due to the similarities of this disorder to OCD. Cognitive behavioral therapy may have some efficacy. Coexisting psychiatric conditions, such as a mood disorder, should be treated. Surgical repair of the "defect" is rarely successful.

# Factitious Disorder

I. **DSM-IV Criteria**
   A. Intentional production of physical or psychological symptoms.
   B. The patients motivation is to assume the sick role.
   C. External motives (financial gain) are absent.

II. **Clinical Features of Factitious Disorder**
   A. Identity disturbance and dependent and narcissistic traits are frequent. Patients with physical symptoms often have histories of many surgeries and hospitalizations.
   B. Patients are able to provide a detailed history and describe symptoms of a particular disease and may intentionally produce symptoms (eg, use of drugs such as insulin, self-inoculation to produce abscesses). Common coexisting psychological symptoms include depression or factitious psychosis.
   C. Great effort should be made to confirm the facts presented by the patient and confirm the past medical history. An outside informant should be

          sought to provide corroborating information.

## III. Epidemiology of Factitious Disorder
    **A.** Begins in early adulthood.
    **B.** More frequent in men and among health-care workers.

## IV. Classification of Factitious Disorder
    **A.** With predominantly psychological signs and symptoms.
    **B.** With predominantly physical signs and symptoms (also known as Münchhausen Syndrome).
    **C.** With combined psychological and physical symptoms.
    **D.** Factitious disorder by proxy is characterized by the production of feigning of physical signs or symptoms in another person who is under the person's care (typically a child). This is considered to be a form of child abuse.

## V. Differential Diagnosis
    **A. Somatoform Disorders:** Somatoform disorder patients are less willing to undergo medical procedures, such as surgery. Symptoms are not fabricated.
    **B. Malingering:** A recognizable goal for producing symptoms is present.
    **C. Ganser's syndrome** refers to a condition associated with prison inmates who give ridiculous answers to questions (1 + 1 = 5) in an effort to avoid responsibility for their actions.

## VI. Treatment of Factitious Disorder
    **A.** No specific treatment exists, and the prognosis is generally poor.
    **B.** The condition should be recognized early, and needless medical procedures should be prevented. Close collaboration between the medical staff and psychiatrist is recommended.

*References*
References, see page 120.

# Sleep Disorders

## Primary Insomnia

Primary insomnia is characterized by the inability to initiate or maintain sleep.

**I. DSM-IV Criteria**
  **A.** Difficulty initiating or maintaining sleep when there is no known physical or mental condition (including drug related), resulting in significant distress or impairment.
  **B.** The disorder causes significant distress or impairment in social or occupational functioning.
  **C.** The disorder is not due to the effects of medication, drugs of abuse, or a medical condition.

**II. Clinical Features**
  **A.** Anxiety or depression commonly coexist with insomnia.
  **B.** Mood disorders account for less than 50% of insomnia.
  **C.** Schizophrenia is associated with fragmented sleep.

**III. Differential Diagnosis**
  **A.** Dyssomnias, substance abuse, mood, anxiety, or psychotic disorders may present with insomnia.
  **B.** Many medical conditions can cause insomnia including asthma, gastritis, peptic ulcer disease, headaches.
  **C.** Many drugs can disrupt sleep including beta-blockers, calcium channel blockers, steroids, decongestants, nicotine, stimulating antidepressants, thyroid hormones, and bronchodilators.

**IV. Treatment**
  **A.** Temporary use (less than one month) of short-acting benzodiazepines is especially helpful when there is an identifiable precipitant (eg, death of a loved one).
  **B.** Zolpidem (Ambien) and zaleplon (Sonata) have the advantage of achieving hypnotic effects with less tolerance and less daytime sedation.
  **C.** The safety profile of benzodiazepines and benzodiazepine receptor agonists is good; lethal overdose is rare, except when benzodiazepines are taken with alcohol.
  **D.** Zolpidem (Ambien) is a benzodiazepine receptor agonist with a short elimination half-life that is effective in inducing sleep onset and promoting sleep maintenance. Zolpidem is associated with greater residual impairment in memory and psychomotor performance than zaleplon.
  **E.** Zaleplon (Sonata) is a benzodiazepine receptor agonist that is rapidly absorbed ($T_{max}$ = 1 hour) and has a short elimination half-life of one hour. Zaleplon does not impair memory or psychomotor functioning on morning awakening. Zaleplon does not cause residual impairment when the drug is taken in the middle of the night. It can be used at bedtime or after the patient has tried to fall asleep naturally.
  **F.** Eszopiclone (Lunesta) is a benzodiazepine receptor agonist with a 6-hour elimination half-life that is effective in inducing sleep onset and promoting sleep maintenance. Eszopiclone is associated with greater residual impairment in memory and psychomotor performance than zaleplon.

**G. Ramelteon (Rozerem)** binds to melatonin receptors $MT_1$, $MT_2$) and is useful for insomnia characterized by difficulty with sleep onset. It does not have abuse liability nor does it cause cognitive impairment or CNS depression.

**H. Benzodiazepines with long half-lives**, such as flurazepam (Dalmane), may be effective in promoting sleep onset and sustaining sleep. These drugs tend to accumulate and have effects that extend beyond the desired sleep period, resulting in daytime sedation or functional impairment. This can be particularly problematic in the elderly who have reduced metabolic clearance of these medications.

**I. Sedating antidepressants** are sometimes used as an alternative to benzodiazepines or benzodiazepine receptor agonists. Amitriptyline (Elavil), 25-50 mg at bedtime, doxepin (Sinequan) 50 mg, mirtazapine (Remeron) 7.5-15 mg or trazodone (Desyrel), 50-100 mg, are common choices.

**J. Sleep Hygiene**
   1. Encourage patient to keep a consistent pattern of waking, and sleeping at the same time each day.
   2. Avoid large meals before bedtime.
   3. Discontinue stimulant caffeine, alcohol, or nicotine.
   4. Avoid daytime naps.
   5. Engage in regular exercise, but avoid exercise before sleeping.
   6. Allow for a period of relaxation before bedtime (hot bath).

| Agents Used for Insomnia | | | |
|---|---|---|---|
| **Agent** | **Dosage** | **Ave Half-life of Metabolites** | **Comments** |
| Zolpidem (Ambien, Ambien CR) | 5-10 mg qhs 6.25-12.5 mg | 3 hours | Non-benzodiazepine; no daytime hangover. CR provides longer-term action. 6.25 mg dose is recommended for elderly. |
| Zaleplon (Sonata) | 5-10 mg | 1 hour | Non-benzodiazepine; no daytime hangover |
| Eszopiclone (Lunesta) | 1-3 mg | 6 hours | Non-benzodiazepine |
| Triazolam (Halcion) | 0.125-0.25 mg qhs | 2 hours | Short acting; some patients can experience perceptual disturbances |
| Temazepam (Restoril) | 7.5-30 mg qhs | 11 hours | Benzodiazepine |
| Flurazepam (Dalmane) | 15-30 mg qhs | 100 hours, active metabolites long t ½ | Hangover is common. Can accumulate in elderly. Benzodiazepine. |

| Agent | Dosage | Ave Half-life of Metabolites | Comments |
|-------|--------|------------------------------|----------|
| Ramelteon (Rozerem) | 8 mg qhs | metabolite has little activity | Non-benzodiazepine; half-life of ramelteon is 1-2 hours; no abuse liability |
| **Antidepressants** Trazodone (Desyrel) | 25-100mg | Long | Priapism - rare. |
| Doxepin (Sinequan) | 50-100 mg | Long | Anticholinergic side effects |
| Amitriptyline (Elavil) | 25-50 mg | Long | Anticholinergic side effects |
| Mirtazapine (Remeron) | 7.5-15 mg | Long | More sedating at lower doses. |
| **Antihistamines** Diphenhydramine (Benadryl) | 50 mg | NA | Limited efficacy for mild initial insomnia. |

## Primary Hypersomnia

I. **DSM-IV Criteria for Primary Hypersomnia**
   A. Excessive somnolence occurs for one month in the absence of physical or medical condition and is associated with daytime sleepiness.
   B. The disorder causes significant distress or impairment in social or occupational functioning.
   C. The disorder is not due to the effects of medication, drugs of abuse, or a medical condition.
II. **Clinical Features**
   A. Depression often coexists.
   B. Can be associated with autonomic dysfunction.
   C. May be familial.
   D. Sleep architecture is normal.
III. **Differential Diagnosis**
   A. **Substance abuse,** mood, anxiety, or psychotic disorders may present with hypersomnia.
   B. **Atypical depression** and the depressed phase of bipolar illness may present with hypersomnia as an isolated symptom.
IV. **Treatment**. For daytime sleepiness stimulants such as amphetamine or methylphenidate (Ritalin), given in the morning, are useful. Modafinil (Provigil) is a non-amphetamine stimulant approved for treatment of excessive daytime sleepiness associated with narcolepsy. Modafinil is effective at a dosage of 100-200 mg given in the morning.

# Narcolepsy

**I. DSM-IV Criteria for Narcolepsy**
   A. Excessive daytime sleepiness.
   B. Sleep attacks with abnormal manifestations of rapid eye movement sleep during the day. Sleep attacks may be associated with hallucinations, sleep paralysis, sleep onset REM, or cataplexy.
   C. The disorder causes significant distress or impairment in social or occupational functioning.
   D. The disorder is not due to the effects of medication, drugs of abuse, or a medical condition.

**II. Clinical Features**
   A. Social reticence occurs due to fear of having sleep attack. Sudden onset of sleep (cataplexy) can be triggered by strong emotions.
   B. Narcolepsy is often associated with mood disorders, substance abuse, and generalized anxiety disorder.
   C. May be familial (>90% have HLA-DR2).

**III. Differential Diagnosis**: Sleep deprivation, primary hypersomnia, breathing-related disorders, hypersomnia associated with mental disorder, such as depression, substance abuse, or a medical condition.

**IV. Treatment**: Stimulants, such as methylphenidate (Ritalin), 10 mg bid or tid, are sometimes combined with tricyclic antidepressants (Protriptyline 10-20 mg) before bedtime. Modafinil (Provigil) is a non-amphetamine stimulant approved for treatment of excessive daytime sleepiness associated with narcolepsy. Modafinil is effective at a dosage of 200 mg given in the morning.
   A. **Sodium Oxybate (Xyrem)** is a CNS depressant that treats excessive daytime sleepiness and cataplexy associated with narcolepsy. It is also known as GBH and has abuse potential. It comes in a liquid formulation and is titrated to a dose of 6-9 grams/night.

# Breathing-Related Sleep Disorder (Sleep Apnea)

**I. DSM-IV Criteria for Breathing-Related Sleep Disorder**
   A. Sleep disruption leading to daytime sleepiness due to a sleep-related condition.
   B. The disturbance is not due to another mental disorder (eg, depression) or to the effect of drugs of abuse, medication or general medical condition such as arthritis.
   C. The disorder causes significant distress or impairment in social or occupational functioning.

**II. Clinical Features**
   A. Sleep apnea is associated with snoring, restless sleep, memory disturbance, poor concentration, depression, and anxiety disorders.
   B. Nocturnal polysomnography demonstrates apneic episodes, frequent arousals, and decreased slow wave and rapid eye movement sleep.
   C. Apnea can be central due to brain stem dysfunction or obstructive caused by airway obstruction. Obstructive sleep apnea is the most common type.

**III. Differential Diagnosis**: Other Dysomnias, medical conditions and substance abuse or withdrawal may cause sleep disturbances.

**IV. Treatment**

**A.** Nasal continuous positive airway pressure (NCPAP) is the treatment of choice.

**B.** Weight loss, nasal surgery, and uvuloplasty are also indicated if they are contributing to the apnea. Surgical interventions are not consistently effective.

# Circadian Rhythm Sleep Disorder

**I. DSM-IV Criteria for Circadian Rhythm Sleep Disorder**

    **A.** Misalignment between desired and actual sleep periods, which can occur with jet lag or shift work, or can be idiopathic.

    **B.** The disorder causes significant distress or impairment in social or occupational functioning.

    **C.** The disorder is not due to the effects of medication, drugs of abuse, or a medical condition.

**II. Clinical Features**

    **A.** With jet lag and shift work, performance can be impaired during wakefulness.

    **B.** Mood disorders, such as depression and mania, can be precipitated by sleep deprivation.

**III. Treatment**

    **A.** The body naturally adapts to time shifts within one week.

    **B.** Zolpidem (Ambien) or zaleplon (Sonata) can be used to correct sleep pattern.

    **C.** Melatonin (5-10mg), given at 9:00pm, can also be helpful. Higher doses tend not to be as effective, producing a sustained plasma level rather than a brief "pulse" that serves as a signal.

# Dyssomnias Not Otherwise Specified

**I. Nocturnal Myoclonus (periodic leg movements)**

    **A.** Abrupt contractions of leg muscles.

    **B.** Common in elderly (40%).

    **C.** Results in frequent arousals and daytime somnolence.

    **D.** Standard treatments include L-dopa and benzodiazepines.

**II. Restless Legs Syndrome**

    **A.** Painful or uncomfortable sensations in calves when sitting or lying down.

    **B.** Common in middle age (5%).

    **C.** Massage, benzodiazepines, propranolol, opioids or carbamazepine can be helpful. Clonazepam has been effective in doses of 0.5-2.0mg q hs.

# *Substance-Abuse Disorders*

## General Criteria

**DSM-IV Diagnostic for Criteria Substance-Related Disorders**

**I. Substance Intoxication**
   A. Intoxication is defined as a reversible syndrome that develops following ingestion of a substance.
   B. Significant maladaptive, behavioral or psychological changes occur, such as mood lability, impaired judgement, and impaired social or occupational functioning due to ingestion of the substance.

**II. Substance Abuse**
   A. Substance use has not met criteria for dependence, but has lead to impairment or distress as indicated by at least one of the following during a 12-month period:
      1. Failure to meet work, school, or home obligations.
      2. Substance use during hazardous activities.
      3. Recurrent substance-related legal problems.
      4. Continued use of the substance despite continued social problems.

**III. Substance Dependence**
   A. The diagnosis of substance dependence requires substance use, accompanied by impairment, and the presence of three of the following in a 12-month period:
      1. **Tolerance:** An increased amount of substance is required to achieve the same effect, or a decreased effect results when the same amount is used.
      2. **Withdrawal:** A characteristic withdrawal syndrome occurs, or the substance is used in an effort to avoid withdrawal symptoms.
      3. The substance is used in increasingly larger amounts or over a longer period of time than desired.
      4. The patient attempts or desires to decrease use.
      5. A significant amount of time is spent obtaining, using, or recovering from the substance.
      6. Substance use results in a decreased amount of time spent in social, occupational, or recreational activities.
      7. The patient has knowledge that the substance use is detrimental to his health, but that knowledge does not deter continued use.

**IV. Substance Withdrawal**
   A. A substance-specific syndrome develops after cessation or reduction in the amount of substance used.
   B. The syndrome causes clinically significant distress or impairment.
   C. Symptoms are not due to a medical condition or other mental disorder.

**V. Substance-Induced Disorders**
   A. Substance-induced disorders include delirium, dementia, persisting amnestic disorder, psychotic disorder, mood disorder, anxiety disorder, sexual dysfunction, and sleep disorder.
   B. Diagnosis requires meeting criteria for specific disorder with evidence that substance intoxication and not another condition (medical disorder) has caused the symptoms.

## VI. Clinical Evaluation of Substance Abuse

**A.** The physician should determine the amount and frequency of alcohol or other drug use in the past month, week, and day. For alcohol use, the number of days per week alcohol is consumed, and the quantity consumed should be determined.

**B. Effects of Substance Use on the Patient's Life**

1. **Family Manifestations.** Family dysfunction, marital problems, divorce, physical abuse and violence.
2. **Social Manifestations.** Alienation and loss of friends, gravitation toward others with similar lifestyle.
3. **Work or School Manifestations.** Decline in work or school performance, frequent job changes, frequent absences, requests for work excuses.
4. **Legal Manifestations.** Arrests for disturbing the peace or driving while intoxicated, stealing, drug dealing, prostitution, motor vehicle accidents.
5. **Financial Manifestations.** Irresponsible borrowing or owing money, selling of possessions.

## VII. Physical Examination

**A.** Intranasal cocaine use may cause damaged nasal mucosa. IV drug abuse may be associated with injection-site scars and bacterial endocarditis.

**B.** Nystagmus is often seen in abusers of sedatives, hypnotics, or cannabis. Mydriasis (dilated pupils) is often seen in persons under the influence of stimulants or hallucinogens, or in withdrawal from opiates. Miosis (pinpoint pupils) is a classic sign of opioid intoxication.

**C.** The patient should be assessed for the withdrawal symptoms, such as an enlarged liver, spider angioma, impaired liver function, ascites, and signs of poor nutrition or presence of findings due to chronic alcohol use.

## VIII. Laboratory Evaluation of Substance Abuse

**A.** A UA, CBC, chemistry panel, liver function tests, thyroid hormone, and serology should be completed on all patients.

**B.** Impaired liver function and hematologic abnormalities are common.

**C.** Illicit drugs may be detected in blood and urine.

**D.** When risk factors are present, HIV and Hepatitis C testing should be done.

## Specific Substance-induced Disorders

| | Intoxication delirium | Withdrawal delirium | Dementia | Psychotic disorder | Mood disorder | Anxiety disorder | Sexual dysfunction | Sleep disorder |
|---|---|---|---|---|---|---|---|---|
| Alcohol | I | W | P | IW | IW | IW | I | IW |
| Amphetamine | I | | | I | IW | | I | IW |
| Caffeine | | | | | | I | | I |
| Cannabis | I | | | I | | I | | |
| Cocaine | I | | | I | IW | IW | I | IW |
| Hallucinogens | I | | | I | I | I | | |
| Inhalants | I | | P | I | I | I | | |
| Opioids | I | | | I | I | | I | IW |
| PCP | I | | | I | I | I | | |
| Sedative hypnotic | I | W | P | IW | IW | W | I | IW |

I = intoxication  W = withdrawal  P = persisting

# Substance-Related Disorders

## I. Alcohol, Sedatives, Hypnotics, and Anxiolytics

### A. Diagnostic Criteria for Intoxication
1. Behavioral and psychological changes are present.
2. **One or more of the following:** slurred speech, incoordination, unsteady gait, nystagmus, impaired attention or memory, stupor or coma.

### B. Clinical Features of Intoxication
1. Amnesia is often present.
2. Behavioral disinhibition (aggressive or sexual activity) is a common finding.

### C. Addiction
1. Tolerance develops to sedative effects.
2. Tolerance to brainstem depressant effects develops more slowly. As users require higher doses to achieve a "high," the risk for respiratory depression is increased.

### D. Withdrawal from Alcohol and other Sedatives
1. Detoxification may be necessary after prolonged use of central nervous system depressants, or when there are signs of abuse or addiction.
2. Sedatives associated with withdrawal syndromes include alcohol, benzodiazepines, barbiturates, and chloral hydrate.

### E. Detoxification of Patients Dependent on Alcohol, Sedatives or Hypnotics
1. Provide a supervised stepwise dose reduction of the drug or substitute a cross-tolerant, longer-acting substance (diazepam), which has less risk of severe withdrawal symptoms.
2. The cross-tolerated drug is given in gradually tapering doses. To prevent withdrawal symptoms, the dose of medication should be reduced gradually over 1-2 weeks.

## II. Cocaine

### A. Diagnostic Criteria for Intoxication
1. Psychological or behavioral changes, such as euphoria, hyperactivity, hypersexuality, grandiosity, anxiety, or impaired judgement, are present.
2. **Two or more of the following:** tachycardia or bradycardia, mydriasis (dilated pupils), high or low blood pressure, chills or perspiration, nausea or vomiting, weight loss, agitation or retardation, weakness, arrhythmias, confusion, seizures, coma, respiratory depression, dyskinesias, or dystonia.

### B. Clinical Features of Cocaine Abuse
1. Irritability, poor concentration, insomnia, and personality change are common. Intoxication can result in euphoria, impulsive behavior, poor judgement, and perceptual disturbances.
2. Physical sequelae include seizures, nasal congestion and bleeding, cerebral infarcts, and arrhythmias.
3. Chronic use is associated with paranoid ideation, aggressive behavior, depression, and weight loss.

### C. Addiction.
Psychological dependence is frequent. Tolerance develops with repeated use.

### D. Withdrawal
is characterized by depression, hypersomnia, anhedonia,

anxiety, fatigue, and an intense craving for the drug; withdrawal generally remits in 2-5 days. Drug craving may last for months.

### E. Treatment
1. Hospitalization is sometimes required during the withdrawal phase of treatment because of the intense craving.
2. Clonidine, amantadine, carbamazepine and tricyclic antidepressants (desipramine), may decrease craving and are often adjuncts to treatment.

## III. Opioids

### A. Diagnostic Criteria for Intoxication
1. Behavioral or psychological changes, such as euphoria, followed by dysphoria, psychomotor retardation, impaired judgement, or impaired social or occupational functioning.
2. Pinpoint pupils (meiosis).
3. One of the following: drowsiness, coma, slurred speech, or impairment in attention or memory.

### B. Clinical Features of Opioid Abuse
1. Initial euphoria is followed by apathy, dysphoria, and psychomotor retardation. Overdose can result in coma, respiratory depression, and death.
2. IV use is associated with risk of AIDS, skin abscesses, and bacterial endocarditis.

### C. Addiction. Tolerance and dependence develops rapidly.

### D. Withdrawal
1. Intensity of the withdrawal syndrome is greatest with opiates that have a short half-life, such as heroin. Heroin withdrawal begins eight hours after the last use, peaks in 2-3 days and can last up to 10 days.
2. Diagnosis of withdrawal requires the presence of three or more of the following: dysphoria, nausea, vomiting, muscle aches, lacrimation, rhinorrhea, mydriasis, piloerection, sweating, diarrhea, yawning, fever, and insomnia.

### E. Treatment of Heroin Addiction
1. For patients with respiratory compromise an airway should be established and naloxone (0.4 mg IV) should be given immediately.
2. Withdrawal symptoms can be managed with methadone (20-80 mg/day) buprenorphine or clonidine (given orally or by patch). Clonidine (0.1-0.3 mg qid) is effective and is usually used as a first-line treatment of withdrawal. (Also see Opiate Dependance, page 10.)

## IV. Phencyclidine Abuse

### A. Diagnostic Criteria for Intoxication
1. Behavioral changes.
2. At least two of the following: nystagmus, hypertension or tachycardia, slurred speech, ataxia, decreased pain sensitivity, muscle rigidity, seizure or coma, hyperacusis.

### B. Clinical Features of Phencyclidine Abuse
1. Behavior changes include violence, belligerence, hyperactivity, catatonia, psychosis, anxiety, impairment of attention or memory, difficulty communicating.
2. Perceptual disturbances include paranoia, hallucinations, and confusion.
3. **Physical Examination:** Fever, diaphoresis, mydriasis.
4. **Toxicology:** PCP can be detected in urine for up to 5 days after

        ingestion.
- **C. Addiction:** No evidence of physical dependence occurs, but tolerance to the effects can occur.
- **D. Withdrawal:** Signs of depression can occur during withdrawal.
- **E. Treatment of Phencyclidine Abuse**
    1. Benzodiazepines are the treatment of choice (lorazepam 2-4 mg PO, IM or IV).
    2. Psychosis is often refractory to treatment with antipsychotics. Haloperidol (Haldol [2-4 mg IM/PO]) every two hours can be used, but drugs with anticholinergic side effects (phenothiazines) should be avoided due to the intrinsic anticholinergic effects of PCP.
    3. Medical support is required if the patient is unconscious.

## V. Amphetamine/Methamphetamine (Speed, Crystal, Crank)

- **A. Diagnostic Criteria for Amphetamine Intoxication**
    1. Behavioral or psychological changes such as euphoria, rapid speech, hyperactivity, hypervigilance, agitation, or irritability.
- **B. Clinical Features**
    1. Euphoria and increased energy is common in new users.
    2. Development of delusions or hallucinations are not unusual in chronic heavy users.
- **C. Addiction:** Physical tolerance develops, requiring increasing doses to achieve usual effect. Psychological dependence is frequent.
- **D. Amphetamine Withdrawal**
    1. Generally resolves in one week and is associated with increased appetite, vivid dreaming, fatigue, anxiety, hypersomnia, insomnia, psychomotor agitation or retardation.
    2. Depression and suicidal ideation can develop.
- **E. Treatment**
    1. Antipsychotics can be used if psychosis is present.
    2. Benzodiazepines such as diazepam or lorazepam may also help calm the patient.

## VI. Nicotine

- **A. Intoxication** does not occur.
- **B. Clinical Features**
    1. Craving is often prominent.
- **C. Addiction:** Tolerance develops rapidly.
- **D. Diagnostic Criteria for Withdrawal**
    1. After abrupt cessation or reduction in the amount of nicotine used, four or more of the following occur within 24 hours: dysphoria, insomnia, irritability, anxiety, poor concentration, restlessness, decreased heart rate, increased appetite.
- **E. Treatment**
    1. Nicorette gum or nicotine transdermal patches relieve withdrawal symptoms. Patients should be prescribed a regimen that provides a tapering dose over a period of weeks.

| Treatments for Smoking Cessation | | |
| --- | --- | --- |
| Drug | Dosage | Comments |
| Nicotine gum (Nicorette) | 2- or 4-mg piece/30 min | Available OTC; poor compliance |
| Nicotine patch (Habitrol, Nicoderm CQ) *other OTC brands available | 1 patch/d for 6-12 weeks, then taper for 4 week | Available OTC; local skin reactions |
| Nicotine nasal spray (Nicotrol NS) | 1-2 doses/h for 6-8 weeks | Rapid nicotine delivery; nasal irritation initially |
| Nicotine inhaler (Nicotrol Inhaler) | 6-16 cartridges/d for 12 weeks | Mimics smoking behavior; provides low doses of nicotine |
| Bupropion (Zyban) | 150 mg/day for 3 d, then titrate to 300 mg | Treatment initiated 2 weeks before quit day; contra-indicated with seizures, anorexia, heavy alcohol use |

**F. Nicotine nasal spray (Nicotrol NS)** is available by prescription and is a good choice for heavy smokers or patients who have failed treatment with nicotine gum or patch. It delivers a high level of nicotine, similar to smoking. The spray is used 6-8 weeks, at 1-2 doses per hour (one puff in each nostril). Tapering over about six weeks.

**G. Nicotine inhaler (Nicotrol Inhaler)** delivers nicotine orally via inhalation from a plastic tube. It is available by prescription and has a success rate of 28%, similar to nicotine gum.

**H. Bupropion (Zyban)**
  1. Bupropion is appropriate for patients who have been unsuccessful using nicotine replacement. Bupropion reduces withdrawal symptoms and can be used in conjunction with nicotine replacement therapy. The treatment is associated with reduced weight gain. Bupropion is contraindicated with a history of seizures, anorexia, heavy alcohol use, or head trauma.
  2. Bupropion is started at a dose of 150 mg daily for three days, then increased to 300 mg daily for two weeks before the patient stops smoking. Bupropion is then continued for three months. When a nicotine patch is added to this regimen, the abstinence rates increase to 50% compared with 32% when only the patch is used.

*References*
References, see page 120.

# Cognitive Disorders

# Delirium

I. **DSM-IV Diagnostic Criteria for Delirium**
   A. Disturbance of consciousness with reduced ability to focus, sustain or shift attention.
   B. The change in cognition or perceptual disturbance is not due to dementia.
   C. The disturbance develops over a short period of time (hours to days) and fluctuates during the course of the day.
   D. There is clinical evidence that the disturbance is caused by a general medical condition and/or substance use or withdrawal.

II. **Clinical Features of Delirium**
   A. Delirium is characterized by impairments of consciousness, awareness of environment, attention and concentration. Many patients are disoriented and display disorganized thinking. A fluctuating clinical presentation is the hallmark of the disorder, and the patient may have moments of lucidity during the course of the day.
   B. Perceptual disturbances may take the form of misinterpretations, illusions or frank hallucinations. The hallucinations are most commonly visual, but other sensory modalities can also be misperceived.
   C. Sleep-wake cycle disturbances are common, and psychomotor agitation can be severe, resulting in pulling out of IVs and catheters, falling, and combative behavior. The quietly delirious patient may reduce fluid and food intake without overtly displaying agitated behavior.
   D. Failure to report use of medications or substance abuse is a common cause of withdrawal delirium in hospitalized patients. Infection and medication interaction or toxicity is a common cause of delirium in the elderly.
   E. Injuries may occur when the patient is delirious and agitated and unrecognized delirium may result in permanent cognitive impairment.
   F. The incidence of delirium in hospitalized patients is 10-15%, with higher rates in the elderly. Other patients at risk include those with CNS disorders, substance abusers, and HIV-positive patients.
   G. Post-discharge morbidity and mortality is higher in patients who experience delirium compared to those who do not.

III. **Classification of Delirium**
   A. Delirium due to a general medical condition (specify which condition).
   B. Delirium due to substance intoxication (specify which substance).
   C. Delirium due to a substance withdrawal (specify which substance).
   D. Delirium due to a multiple etiologies (specify which conditions).
   E. Delirium not otherwise specified (unknown etiology or due to other causes such as sensory deprivation).

IV. **Differential Diagnosis of Delirium**
   A. **Dementia**
      1. Dementia is the most common disorder that must be distinguished from delirium. The major difference between dementia and delirium is that demented patients are alert without the disturbance of consciousness characteristic of delirious patients.

    **2.** Information from family or caretakers is helpful in determining whether there was a pre-existing dementia.

  **B. Psychotic Disorders and Mood Disorders with Psychotic Features.** Delirium can be distinguished from psychotic symptoms by the abrupt development of cognitive deficits including disturbance of consciousness. In delirium, there should be some evidence of an underlying medical or substance-related condition.

  **C. Malingering.** Patients with malingering lack objective evidence of a medical or substance-related condition.

## V. Treatment of Delirium

  **A.** Most cases of delirium are treated by correcting the underlying condition.

  **B.** Agitation, confusion, and perceptual disturbances may require treatment with haloperidol (Haldol), 1-2 mg given every 4-8 hours. Haloperidol is the only antipsychotic available in IV form. Intravenous administration may be necessary in medically ill patients. Haloperidol may also be given IM.

  **C.** If patients are willing to take oral medication, small doses of the sedating, low-potency medication quetiapine (Seroquel) 12.5-25 mg every 4-8 hours can be very effective. Monitoring of heart rate and blood pressure is necessary in patients receiving more than two doses per day. Parenteral forms of ziprasidone (Geodon) and olanzapine (Zyprexa) may have a role in managing delirium.

  **D.** Agitation can also be treated with lorazepam (Ativan), 1-2 mg every 2-6 hours PO, IM or IV. Lorazepam is safe in the elderly and those patients with compromised renal or hepatic function. It should be used cautiously in patients with respiratory dysfunction. It may cause increased confusion.

  **E.** A quiet environment with close observation should be provided. Physical restraints may be necessary to prevent injury to self or others.

# Dementia

## I. DSM-IV Diagnostic Criteria for Dementia

  **A.** The development of multiple cognitive deficits manifested by:

    **1.** Memory impairment.

    **2. One or more of the following:**

      **a.** Aphasia (language disturbance).

      **b.** Apraxia (impaired ability to carry out purposeful movement, especially the use of objects).

      **c.** Agnosia (failure to recognize or identify objects).

      **d.** Disturbance in executive functioning (abstract thinking, planning and carrying out tasks).

  **B.** The cognitive deficits cause significant social and occupational impairment and represent a significant decline from a previous level of functioning.

  **C.** The deficits are not the result of delirium.

## II. Clinical Features of Dementia

A. The memory impairment involves difficulty in learning new material and/or forgetting previously learned material. Early signs may consist of losing belongings or getting lost more easily.

B. Once the dementia is well established, patients may have great difficulty performing activities of daily living such as bathing, dressing, cooking, or shopping.

C. Poor insight and impaired judgment are common features of dementia.

   1. Patients are often unaware of their deficits.
   2. Patients may overestimate their ability to safely carry out specific tasks.
   3. Disinhibition can lead to poor social judgment, such as making inappropriate comments.

D. Psychiatric symptoms are common and patients frequently manifest symptoms of anxiety, depression, and sleep disturbance.

E. Paranoid delusions (especially accusations that others are stealing items) and hallucinations (especially visual) are common.

F. Delirium is frequently superimposed upon dementia because these patients are more sensitive to the effects of medications and physical illness.

## III. Epidemiology of Dementia

A. The prevalence of dementia increases with age. Three percent of patients over 65 years old have dementia, but after age 85, 20% of the population is affected.

B. Alzheimer's type dementia is the most common type of dementia, comprising 50-60% of all cases. Vascular dementia is the second most common cause of dementia, accounting for 13% of all cases.

## IV. Classification of Dementia

### A. Alzheimer's Type Dementia

   1. The patient meets basic diagnostic criteria for dementia but also:
      a. Gradual onset and continued cognitive decline.
      b. Cognitive deficits are not due to another medical condition or substance.
      c. Symptoms are not caused by another psychiatric disorder.
   2. Alzheimer's Disease is further classified as:
      a. Early or late onset.
      b. With delirium, delusions, depressed mood, or uncomplicated.
   3. The average life expectancy after onset of illness is 8-10 years.

### B. Vascular Dementia (previously Multi-Infarct Dementia)

   1. The patient meets basic diagnostic criteria for dementia but also has:
      a. Focal neurological signs and symptoms or laboratory evidence of cerebrovascular disease (eg, multiple infarctions on MRI scan).
      b. Vascular dementia is further classified as with delirium, delusions, depressed mood, or uncomplicated.
      c. Unlike Alzheimer's disease, changes in functioning may be abrupt, and the long-term course tends to have a stepwise pattern. Deficits are highly variable depending on the location of the vascular lesions, leaving some cognitive functions intact.

### C. Dementia Due to Other General Medical Conditions

   1. Meets basic diagnostic criteria for dementia, but there must also be evidence that symptoms are the direct physiological consequence of a general medical condition.

2. **AIDS-Related Dementia**
   a. Dementia caused by the effect of the HIV virus on the brain.
   b. Clinical presentation includes psychomotor retardation, forgetfulness, apathy, impaired problem solving, flat affect, social withdrawal.
   c. Frank psychosis may be present.
   d. Neurological symptoms are frequently present.
3. **Dementia Caused by Head Trauma**. Dementia caused by head trauma usually does not progress. The one notable exception is dementia pugilistica, which is caused by repeated trauma (eg, boxing).
4. **Dementia Caused by Parkinson's Disease.** Dementia occurs in 40-60% of patients with Parkinson's disease. The dementia is often exaggerated by the presence of major depression.
5. **Dementia Caused by Huntington's Disease**
   a. Dementia is an inevitable outcome of this disease.
   b. Initially, language and factual knowledge may be relatively preserved, while memory, reasoning, and executive function are more seriously impaired.
   c. Occasionally, dementia can precede the onset of motor symptoms.
6. **Dementia Caused by Pick's Disease**
   a. The early phases of the disease are characterized by disinhibition, apathy, and language abnormalities because Pick's disease affects the frontal and temporal lobes.
   b. Later stages of the illness may by clinically similar to Alzheimer's disease. Brain imaging studies usually reveal frontal and/or temporal atrophy.
7. **Dementia Caused by Creutzfeldt-Jakob Disease**
   a. Creutzfeldt-Jacob disease is a subacute spongiform encephalopathy caused by a prion.
   b. The clinical triad consists of dementia, involuntary myoclonic movements, and periodic EEG activity.
8. **Lewy Body Dementia**
   a. Characterized by decline in cognition along with fluctuating levels of attention and alertness. Recurrent, well-formed visual hallucinations are also common.
   b. Lewy body dementia is associated with repeated falls, transient loss of consciousness, syncope, neuroleptic sensitivity, delusions and hallucinations.
D. **Substance-Induced Persisting Dementia**
   1. **Meets basic diagnostic criteria for Dementia but also:**
      a. The deficits persists beyond the usual duration of substance intoxication or withdrawal.
      b. There is evidence that the deficits are related to the persisting effects of substance use (specify which drug or medication).
   2. When drugs of abuse are involved, most patients have, at some time in their lives, met criteria for substance dependence.
   3. Clinical presentation is that of a typical dementia. Occasionally patients will improve mildly after the substance use has been discontinued, but most display a progressive downhill course.
E. **Dementia Due to Multiple Etiologies.** This diagnosis is applicable when multiple disorders are responsible for the dementia.

| General Medical Conditions That Can Cause Dementia | |
|---|---|
| **Vascular**<br>Multiple infarcts<br>Subacute bacterial endocarditis<br>Congestive heart failure<br>Collagen vascular diseases (eg, SLE) | **Neurological**<br>Normal pressure hydrocephalus<br>Huntington's disease<br>Parkinson's disease<br>Pick's disease<br>Brain tumor<br>Multiple sclerosis<br>Head trauma<br>Cerebral anoxia/hypoxia<br>Seizures |
| **Nutritional**<br>Folate deficiency<br>Vitamin $B_{12}$ deficiency<br>Thiamine deficiency (Wernicke<br>Korsakoff syndrome)<br>Pellagra | **Metabolic and Endocrine**<br>Hypothyroidism<br>Hyperparathyroidism<br>Pituitary insufficiency<br>Diabetes<br>Hepatic encephalopathy<br>Uremia<br>Porphyria<br>Wilson's disease |
| **Infections**<br>HIV<br>Cryptococcal meningitis<br>Encephalitis<br>Sarcoid<br>Neurosyphilis<br>Creutzfeldt-Jakob disease | **Toxicity**<br>Heavy metals<br>Intracranial radiation<br>Post-infectious encephalomyelitis<br>Chronic alcoholism<br>Industrial chemicals |

## V. Differential Diagnosis of Dementia
### A. Delirium
   1. Delirium is the most common disorder that may mimic dementia. Differentiation of delirium from dementia can be difficult because demented individuals are prone to developing a superimposed delirium.
   2. Demented patients are alert, whereas, delirious patients have an altered level of consciousness. Delirious patients demonstrate an acutely fluctuating clinical course, whereas demented patients display a stable, slowly progressive, downhill course.
### B. Amnestic Disorder is characterized by isolated memory disturbance, without the cognitive deficits seen in dementia.
### C. Major Depressive Disorder
   1. Both dementia and depression may present with apathy, poor concentration, and impaired memory. Cognitive deficits due to a mood disorder may appear to be dementia, and this is referred to as "pseudodementia."
   2. Differentiation of dementia from depression can be difficult, especially in the elderly. Demented patients are often also depressed. In depression, the mood symptoms should precede the development of cognitive deficits and in dementia, and the cognitive symptoms should precede the depression.
   3. A medical evaluation to rule out treatable causes of dementia or medical causes of depression should be completed.

    **4.** If the distinction between dementia and depression remains unclear, a trial of antidepressants is warranted. If the depression is super-imposed on the dementia, treatment of the depression will improve the functional level of the patient.

## VI. Clinical Evaluation of Dementia

**A.** All patients presenting with cognitive deficits should be evaluated to determine the etiology of the dementia. Some causes of dementia are treatable and reversible.

**B.** A medical and psychiatric history and a physical examination and psychiatric assessment, with special attention to the neurological exam, should be completed.

## VII. Laboratory Evaluation of Dementia

**A.** Complete blood chemistry.

**B.** CBC with differential.

**C.** Thyroid function tests.

**D.** Urinalysis.

**E.** Drug screen.

**F.** Serum levels of all measurable medications.

**G.** Vitamin $B_{12}$ level.

**H.** Heavy metal screen.

**I.** Serological studies (VDRL or MHA-TP).

**J.** EKG.

**K.** Chest X-ray.

**L.** EEG.

**M.** Brain Imaging (CT, MRI) is indicated if there is a suspicion of CNS pathology, such as a mass lesion or vascular event.

## VIII. Treatment of Dementia

**A.** Any underlying medical conditions should be corrected. The use of CNS depressants and anticholinergic medications should be minimized. Patients function best if highly stimulating environments are avoided.

**B.** The family and/or caretakers should receive psychological support. Support groups, psychotherapy, and day-care centers are helpful.

**C. Treatment of Alzheimer's Disease**

    **1. Donepezil (Aricept), Galantamine (Reminyl) and Rivastigmine (Exelon)** are the drugs of choice for improving cognitive functioning in Alzheimer's dementia. They work by central, reversible inhibition of acetylcholinesterase thereby increasing CNS levels of acetylcholine. It may slow progress of the disease.

        **a.** Beginning dose is 5 mg qhs for donepezil, which (after 4-6 weeks) may be increased to 10 mg qhs if necessary. Donepezil has no reported hepatic toxicity or significant drug interactions. Side effects include GI upset or diarrhea.

        **b.** Galantamine (Reminyl)is initiated at 4.0 mg po bid for 4 weeks, then increased to 8.0 mg po bid if tolerated for 4 weeks, and then up to 12 mg po bid.

        **c.** Rivastigmine (Exelon) dosing is begun at 1.5 mg bid, increased to 4.5 mg bid and then 6.0 mg bid at two-week intervals. Efficacy is greatest at the higher dose. The most common side effects are nausea, diarrhea and syncope. GI side effects are reduced by coadministration with food.

    **2. Tacrine (Cognex)** is a less-specific esterase inhibitor that requires monitoring of AST and SLT levels. Tacrine is not used due to its hepatotoxicity.

3. **Memantine (Namenda)** is a noncompetitive antagonist of the N-methyl-D-aspartate (NMDA) receptor indicated for moderate-to-severe dementia. Memantine may be used in conjunction with an acetyl-cholinesterase inhibitor. Dosing is 5 mg po q am, increased by 5 mg/week up to 10 mg po bid.

4. **Vitamin E.** Vitamin E and selegiline (Deprenyl) may also have a role in slowing the progression of dementia.

## D. Treatment of Vascular Dementia

1. Hypertension must be controlled.
2. Aspirin may be indicated to reduce thrombus formation.

## E. Agitation and Aggression

1. **Pharmacotherapy:** The following agents have significant efficacy in reducing agitation and aggression in dementia.

   a. **Atypical Antipsychotics**

   i. **Quetiapine (Seroquel)** 12.5-25 mg po qhs with an increase of 12.5 to 25 mg every 1-3 days if needed to an average dose of 25-200 mg/day and a maximum dose of 400-600 mg/day.

   ii. **Risperidone (Risperdal),** beginning at 0.25-0.5 mg qhs with an average dose of 0.5-2 mg day, is especially effective for agitation associated with psychotic symptoms such as paranoia.

   iii. **Olanzapine (Zyprexa),** beginning at 2.5 mg qhs with an average dose of 2.5-7.5 mg qhs with an average dose of 2.5-7.5 mg qhs, also reduces agitation in dementia.

   iv. **Ziprasidone (Geodon)** 20 mg po bid with increases of 20 mg every 1-3 days as needed with maximum daily dose of 80 mg po bid.

   v. **Aripiprazole (Abilify)** 2.5-5 mg po qhs up to 10 mg if necessary.

   vi. **Haloperidol (Haldol)** may be used if atypical antipsychotics are ineffective or poorly tolerated. Dose range is 0.5-5 mg/day given qhs or bid.

   vii. **Divalproex (Depakote)** at a dosage of 10 mg/kg/day (250-1250 mg/day bid) is effective and well tolerated by many demented patients. Serum levels should be maintained between 25-75 mg/mL.

   viii. There have been reports of increased risk of CVA in the elderly with risperidone, olanzapine and aripiprazole, prompting the FDA to issue a general warning for the entire class of atypicals.

   ix. **Buspirone (BuSpar)** beginning at 5 mg bid with a final dose of 30-50 mg/day in bid or tid dosing. Buspirone has few side effects and no significant drug interactions. Several weeks are required to achieve full benefit. Most commonly used as an adjunct to antipsychotics.

   x. **Trazodone (Desyrel)** beginning at 25-50 mg qhs with an average dose of 50-200 mg/day. Most commonly used as an adjunct.

   xi. **Lorazepam (Ativan),** 0.5-1.0 mg q 4 hours prn, can provide rapid relief, but it is not recommended for long-term use because of ataxia, further memory impairment, and potential for disinhibition and physical dependence.

**F. Psychosis**
1. High-potency typical antipsychotics, such as haloperidol or fluphen-azine, can be effective at very low doses. Atypical antipsychotics are also effective, often at much lower doses than used in patients with primary psychosis.
2. Dosage increases should proceed with caution. The elderly are prone to adverse effects due to serum level accumulation including over-sedation and hypotension.

**G. Depression**
1. SSRIs are first-line antidepressants in the elderly. Venlafaxine (Effexor XR [75 mg to 225 mg]), bupropion (Wellbutrin), mirtazapine (Remeron) and duloxetine (Cymbalta) may also be used if SSRIs are ineffective.
2. Tricyclic antidepressants should be avoided in patients with dementia because of their cardiovascular and anticholinergic effects.

***References***
References, see page 120.

# Mental Disorders Due to a Medical Condition

I. **DSM-IV Diagnostic Criteria for Mental Disorder Due to a Medical Condition**
   A. There is evidence from the history, physical examination, or laboratory studies that the symptoms are a direct physiological consequence of a general medical condition.
   B. The disturbance is not better accounted for by another mental disorder.
   C. The disturbance is not caused by delirium.

II. **Psychotic Disorder Caused by a General Medical Condition**
   A. **Diagnostic Criteria.** The patient meets the criteria for a mental disorder due to a general medical condition and there are prominent hallucinations or delusions.
   B. **Clinical Features of Psychotic Disorder Due to a General Medical Condition**
      1. Hallucinations caused by a medical condition include visual, olfactory and tactile elements more often than in primary psychotic disorders.
      2. Temporal Lobe Epilepsy is a common medical condition associated with olfactory hallucinations. Somatic and persecutory delusions are the most common types of delusions associated with a medical condition.

| Common Disorders Associated with Psychosis | |
|---|---|
| Addison's disease | Lupus |
| CNS infections | Multiple sclerosis |
| CNS neoplasms | Myxedema |
| CNS trauma | Pancreatitis |
| Cushing's disease | Pellagra |
| Delirium | Pernicious anemia |
| Dementias | Porphyria |
| Folic acid deficiency | Temporal lobe epilepsy |
| Huntington's chorea | Thyrotoxicosis |

   C. **Differential Diagnosis of Psychotic Disorder Due to a General Medical Condition**
      1. **Primary Psychotic Disorders**
         a. The onset of illness in a primary psychotic disorder is usually earlier (before age 35), with symptoms beginning prior to the onset of the medical illness.
         b. Complex auditory hallucinations are more characteristic of primary psychotic disorders. Non-auditory hallucinations (eg, tactile hallucinations) are more commonly seen in general medical conditions.
      2. **Substance-Induced Psychotic Disorder**
         a. When psychosis is associated with recent or prolonged substance use, withdrawal from a substance is the likely cause. Blood or urine screens for suspected substances may be helpful in establishing this diagnosis.

      **b. Substances that can cause psychosis:** anticholinergics, steroids, amphetamines, cocaine, hallucinogens, L-dopa, and disulfiram.

**D. Treatment of Psychotic Disorder Due to a General Medical Condition**
  1. The underlying medical conditions should be corrected.
  2. A trial of antipsychotic medication may be necessary to manage symptoms while the patient's medical condition is being treated.

## III. Mood Disorder Due to a General Medical Condition

**A. Diagnostic Criteria.** Meets criteria for a mental disorder due to a general medical condition, and the presence of a prominent and persistent mood disturbance characterized by either or both of the following:
  1. With depressed mood or lack of pleasure in most, if not all, activities.
  2. Elevated, expansive, or irritable mood.

**B. Clinical Features of Mood Disorder Due to a General Medical Condition**
  1. The mood symptoms cannot be a merely psychological reaction to being ill.
  2. **Subtypes include:**
    a. Mood disorder due to a general medical condition with depressive features.
    b. Mood disorder due to a general medical condition with major depressive-like episode.
    c. Mood disorder due to a general medical condition with manic features.
    d. Mood disorder due to a general medical condition with mixed features.

| Common Diseases and Disorders Associated with Depressive Syndromes | |
|---|---|
| Addison's disease | Infectious hepatitis |
| AIDS | Influenza |
| Anemia | Lupus |
| Asthma | Malignancies |
| Chronic infection (mononucleosis, tuberculosis) | Malnutrition |
| | Multiple sclerosis |
| Cushing's disease | Porphyria |
| Diabetes | Rheumatoid arthritis |
| Heart failure | Syphilis |
| Hyperthyroidism | Uremia |
| Hypothyroidism | Ulcerative colitis |

**C. Differential Diagnosis of Mood Disorder Due to a General Medical Condition**
  1. **Primary Mood Disorder.** If a clear causative physiological explanation cannot be established between mood symptoms and the medical condition, a primary mood disorder should be diagnosed. Fluctuation of mood symptoms during the course of medical illness is indicative of a disorder due to a medical condition.
  2. **Substance-Induced Mood Disorder**
    a. When there is evidence of recent or prolonged substance use, a substance-induced mood disorder is most likely. Blood or urine screens may be helpful in establishing this diagnosis.
    b. Common substances that can cause depressive syndromes

include antihypertensives, hormones (cortisone, estrogen, progesterone), antiparkinsonian drugs, benzodiazepines, alcohol, chronic use of sympathomimetics, and withdrawal from psychostimulants.

3. **Treatment of Mood Disorder Due to a General Medical Condition.** The underlying medical condition should be corrected.

*References*
References, see page 120.

# Eating Disorders

---

## Anorexia Nervosa

I. **DSM-IV Diagnostic Criteria for Anorexia Nervosa**
   A. The patient refuses to maintain weight above 85% of expected weight for age and height.
   B. Intense fear of weight gain or of being fat, even though underweight.
   C. Disturbance in the perception of ones weight and shape, or denial of seriousness of current low weight.
   D. Amenorrhea for three cycles in post-menarchal females.

II. **Classification of Anorexia Nervosa**
   A. **Restricting Type or Excessive Dieting Type.** Binging or purging are not present.
   B. **Binge-Eating Type or Purging Type.** Regular binging and purging behavior occurs during current episode (purging may be in the form of vomiting, laxative abuse, enema abuse, or diuretic abuse).

III. **Clinical Features of Anorexia Nervosa**
   A. Anorexia nervosa is characterized by obsessive-compulsive features (counting calories, hoarding food), diminished sexual activity, rigid personality, strong need to control ones environment, and social phobia (fear of eating in public). Anorexia nervosa commonly coexists with major depressive disorder.
   B. Two-thirds of patients with anorexia or bulimia nervosa have a history of a major depressive episode.
   C. **Complications of Anorexia Nervosa.** All body systems may be affected, depending on the degree of starvation and the type of purging. Leukopenia and anemia, dehydration, metabolic acidosis (due to laxatives), or alkalosis (due to vomiting), diminished thyroid function, low sex hormone levels, osteoporosis, bradycardia, and encephalopathy are commonly seen.
   D. Physical signs and symptoms may include gastrointestinal complaints, cold intolerance, emaciation, parotid gland enlargement, lanugo hair, hypotension, peripheral edema, poor dentition, and lethargy.

IV. **Epidemiology of Anorexia Nervosa**
   A. Ninety percent of cases occur in females. The prevalence in females is 0.5-1.0%. The disorder begins in early adolescence and is rare after the age of forty. Peak incidences occur at age 14 and at age 18 years.
   B. There is an increased risk in first-degree relatives, and there is a higher concordance rate in monozygotic twins. Patients with a history of hospitalization secondary to anorexia have a 10% mortality rate.

V. **Differential Diagnosis of Anorexia Nervosa**
   A. **Medical Conditions.** Malignancies, AIDS, superior mesenteric artery syndrome (postprandial vomiting due to gastric outlet obstruction) are not associated with a distorted body image nor the desire to lose weight.
   B. **Body Dysmorphic Disorder.** Additional distortions of body image must be present to diagnose this disorder.
   C. **Bulimia Nervosa.** These patients are usually able to maintain weight at or above the expected minimum.

VI. **Laboratory Evaluation of Anorexia Nervosa.** Decreased serum albumin, globulin, calcium, hypokalemia, hyponatremia, anemia, and leukopenia may be present. ECG may show prolonged QT interval or arrhythmias.

## VII. Treatment of Anorexia Nervosa

**A. Pharmacotherapy of Anorexia Nervosa**
1. There are a number of studies demonstrated improvement in anorexia with SSRIs, with fluoxetine (Prozac) having been most commonly used at doses of 20-60 mg per day. However, there are also a number of studies, which showed negative results in anorexia with SSRI treatment.
2. Trials of low-dose antipsychotic medications have been described with varying success in patients with anorexia. Medication-induced weight gain can affect the acceptability of this treatment and hasten non-compliance.

**B.** Psychotherapies include psychodynamic psychotherapy, family therapy, behavioral therapy, and group therapy.

**C.** Specialized treatment programs, including behavioral treatment focusing on weight gain, family psychotherapy, oral intake monitoring with dietary consultation, and pharmacotherapy are effective in motivated patients. Close monitoring of body weight and the general medical condition is warranted.

**D.** Hospitalization may become necessary if weight loss becomes severe or if hypotension, syncope, or cardiac problems develop.

# Bulimia Nervosa

## I. DSM-IV Diagnostic Criteria for Bulimia Nervosa

**A.** The patient engages in recurrent episodes of binging, characterized by eating an excessive amount of food within a two-hour span and by having a sense of lack of self-control over eating during the episode.

**B.** The patient engages in recurrent compensatory behavior to prevent weight gain (eg, self-induced vomiting, laxative, diuretic, exercise abuse).

**C.** The above occur on the average twice a week for three months.

**D.** The patient's self-evaluation is unduly influenced by body shape and weight.

**E.** The disturbance does not occur exclusively during episodes of anorexia nervosa.

## II. Classification of Bulimia Nervosa

**A. Purging Type Bulimia Nervosa.** The patient regularly makes use of self-induced vomiting, and laxatives.

**B. Nonpurging Type Bulimia Nervosa.** The patient regularly engages in fasting or exercise, but not vomiting or laxatives.

## III. Clinical Features of Bulimia Nervosa

**A.** Unlike anorexia patients, bulimic patients tend to be at or above their expected weight for age. Bulimic patients tend to be ashamed of their behavior and often hide it from their families and physicians.

**B.** There is an increased frequency of affective disorders, substance abuse (30%), and borderline personality disorder (30%) in bulimia patients.

**C.** Purging can be associated with poor dentition (because of acidic damage to teeth). Electrolyte abnormalities (metabolic alkalosis, hypokalemia), dehydration, and various degrees of starvation can occur. Menstrual abnormalities are frequent. Prognosis is generally better than for anorexia nervosa, and death rarely occurs in bulimia.

## IV. Epidemiology of Bulimia Nervosa

A. Bulimia occurs primarily in industrialized countries, and the incidence is 1-3% in adolescent and young adult females and 0.1-0.3% in males.

B. There is a higher incidence of affective disorders in families of patients with bulimia, and obesity is more common.

## V. Differential Diagnosis of Bulimia Nervosa

A. **Binging Purging Type Anorexia Nervosa.** Body weight is less than 85% of expected, and binging and purging behavior occurs.

B. **Atypical Depression.** Overeating occurs in the absence of compensatory purging behaviors, and concern over body shape and weight is not predominant.

C. **Medical Conditions with Disturbed Eating Behaviors.** Loss of control, concern with body shape, and weight are absent.

## VI. Treatment of Bulimia Nervosa

A. The most effective therapy is cognitive behavioral therapy. Psychodynamic group and family therapies are also useful.

B. **Pharmacotherapy of Bulimia Nervosa**

1. Antidepressant medications are useful in the treatment of bulimia nervosa, whether or not accompanied by major depression; symptoms of binging and purging are reduced.

2. SSRIs are most commonly used. Tricyclic antidepressants should be used cautiously, if at all, due to the risk of seizures and cardiotoxicity at high doses or overdose.

3. Bupropion is contraindicated because of the increased risk of seizures in bulimic patients.

### References
References, see page 120.

# Premenstrual Dysphoric Disorder

Premenstrual Dysphoric Disorder (PMDD) is characterized by depressed mood prior to the onset of menses.

## I. DSM-IV Diagnostic Criteria

A. In most menstrual cycles over the past year, 5 or more symptoms were present most of the time in the last week of the luteal phase, began to remit soon after the onset of the follicular phase, and were absent in the week after menses, with at least one of the symptoms being either (1), (2), or (4):

1. Markedly depressed mood, hopelessness, or self-deprecating thoughts.
2. Marked anxiety, tension, feeling "keyed up" or "on edge."
3. Marked affective lability.
4. Persistent and marked anger or irritability or increased interpersonal conflicts.
5. Decreased interest in activities.
6. Subjective sense of difficulty in concentrating.
7. Lethargy, easy fatigability, or marked lack of energy.
8. Marked change in appetite, overeating, or specific food cravings.

9. Hypersomnia or insomnia.

10. A subjective sense of being overwhelmed or out of control.

11. Physical symptoms, such as breast tenderness or swelling, headaches, joint or muscle pain, a sense of "bloating," weight gain.

B. The disturbance markedly interferes with work or school or usual social activities and relationships with others.

C. The disturbance is not merely an exacerbation of the symptoms of another disorder, such as Major Depression, Panic Disorder, Dysthymic Disorder, or a Personality Disorder.

D. Criteria A, B and C must be confirmed by prospective daily ratings during at least two consecutive symptomatic cycles.

## II. Clinical Features of Premenstrual Dysphoric Disorder

A. Patients with PMDD do not experience symptoms in the week following menses. Patients who have continued symptoms after the onset of menses may have another underlying psychiatric disorder.

B. The most severe symptoms of PMDD usually occur in the few days prior to menses. It is uncommon for women with dysmenorrhea to have PMDD and uncommon for women with PMDD to have dysmenorrhea.

## III. Epidemiology of Premenstrual Dysphoric Disorder

A. The prevalence of PMDD ranges from 2-10% in women. Onset usually occurs in the mid to late twenties; however, onset in the teenage years may sometimes occur.

B. Concomitant unipolar depression or bipolar disorder or a family history of affective illness is common in patients with PMDD.

## IV. Differential Diagnosis of Premenstrual Dysphoric Disorder

A. **Premenstrual Syndrome.** Many females experience mild transient affective symptoms around the time of their period. PMDD is diagnosed only when symptoms lead to marked impairment in social and occupational functioning.

B. **Premenstrual Exacerbation of a Current Mood or Anxiety Disorder.** Females with disorders such as dysthymia or generalized anxiety disorder may experience a premenstrual exacerbation of their depressive or anxiety symptoms. These individuals will continue to meet criteria for a mood or anxiety disorder throughout the menstrual cycle; however, patients with PMDD have symptoms only prior to and during menses.

## V. Treatment of Premenstrual Dysphoric Disorder

A. **Antidepressants.** SSRIs, such as fluoxetine (marketed as Sarafem for PMDD), are effective in reducing symptoms of PMDD. The dosage of fluoxetine (Sarafem) is 20 mg per day throughout the month. The dosage may be increased up to 60 mg per day if necessary. Sertraline (Zoloft) is also effective in treating PMDD. Sertraline should be started at 50 mg per day and increased up to 150 mg if necessary. These agents are often effective when given only during the luteal-phase. Other SSRIs are equally effective.

B. **Hormones.** Estrogen, progesterone and triphasic oral contraceptives may improve symptoms of PMDD in some patients.

C. **Spironolactone** may improve physical symptoms, such as bloating.

D. **Anxiolytics.** Alprazolam (Xanax) and buspirone (BuSpar) may have efficacy in treating patients with mild symptoms of anxiety.

E. **Exercise.** Moderate exercise can lead to improvement of physical and emotional symptoms of PMDD.

# Psychiatric Drug Therapy

## Antipsychotic Drug Therapy

### I. Indications for Antipsychotic Drugs

**A.** Antipsychotics (also known as neuroleptics) are indicated for schizo-phrenia, and these agents may be used for other disorders with psychotic features, such as depression and bipolar disorder.

**B.** Antipsychotics are the drugs of choice for brief psychotic disorder, schizophreniform disorder and schizophrenia. They also play a prominent role in the treatment of schizoaffective and bipolar disorder.

**C.** Antipsychotics may be necessary for patients with mood disorders with psychotic features. Brief-to-moderate courses are usually used. These agents often improve functioning in patients with dementia or delirium with psychotic features when given in low doses.

**D.** Antipsychotics are frequently used in the treatment of substance induced psychotic disorders. Low-dose neuroleptics may be useful for the psychotic features of severe personality disorders; however, they should be used with caution and for a brief period of time in these patients.

### II. Selection of an Antipsychotic Agent.
All neuroleptics are equally effective in the treatment of psychosis, with the exception of clozapine, which is more effective for treatment refractory schizophrenia. The newer "atypical" anti-psychotics (risperidone, olanzapine, quetiapine, ziprasidone, and aripiprazole) may be more effective than conventional agents. These newer agents are called atypical because they affect dopamine receptors and also have prominent effects on serotonergic receptors.

**A.** The choice of neuroleptic should be made based on the past history of response to a particular neuroleptic, family history of response, and likelihood of tolerance to side effects.

**B.** At least two weeks of treatment is required before significant antipsychotic effect is achieved. Symptoms will often continue to improve over the following months. The use of more than one antipsychotic agent at a time has not been shown to increase efficacy.

### III. Dosing of Antipsychotic Agents

**A.** Initial treatment for hospitalized patients with acute psychosis usually begins with divided doses of the antipsychotic, such as two to four times per day. Olanzapine (Zyprexa), however, can be initiated with once-a-day dosing. A multiple-dosing schedule can address behavioral issues throughout the day without exposing the patient to the side effects associated with higher doses of medication. This is particularly true of dose-related side effects frequently seen with initiation of medication, such as postural hypotension.

**B.** Outpatients are frequently given once-daily dosing, usually at bedtime. This allows ease of administration and increases compliance.

**C.** Once steady state levels have been achieved (after about five days), the long half-life of most neuroleptics permits once-a-day dosing. Ziprasidone should be given in divided doses.

**D.** Agitated psychotic patients may require additional sedative agents, such as benzodiazepines with antipsychotic medication, until a clinical response occurs.

**IV. Route of Administration**

    **A.** Oral formulations are available for all antipsychotics and some are available in liquid or orally disintegrating form for elderly patients or to increase compliance in patients who "cheek" their medications and later spit them out.

    **B.** Long-acting intramuscular (depot) neuroleptics, such as risperidone (Consta), Haldol decanoate and Prolixin decanoate are useful for non-compliant patients.

        **1.** Haldol decanoate should be started at twenty times the daily oral dose in the first month of treatment, divided into three or four IM injections given over a seven-day period. For example, a patient receiving 20 mg of oral haloperidol per day would be given 400 mg of decanoate. The dose may be reduced by 25% in each of the next two months until the maintenance dose is 200 mg every 30 days.

        **2.** Prolixin decanoate should be started at 25 mg IM every two weeks with the dose adjusted up to 50 mg every two weeks if necessary.

        **3.** Risperdal Consta should be started at 25 mg IM every two weeks with the dose adjusted up to 50 mg every 4 weeks if necessary.

        **4.** Once a patient has received one or two injections, the oral anti-psychotic can be discontinued.

    **C.** Short-acting IM formulations of ziprasidone and olanzapine are available. The recommended dose of IM ziprasidone is 10 mg every 2 hours or 20 mg every 4 hours as required up to a maximum daily dosage of 40 mg. Five to 10 mg of IM olanzapine can be given every 2-4 hours up to a maximum total dose of 30 mg. Haloperidol (Haldol) and chlorpromazine (Thorazine) are often used in IM form to treat acutely agitated psychotic patients. Thorazine is usually given 25-50 mg IM with close monitoring of blood pressure. Haldol 5-10 mg is often given in conjunction with 1-2 mg of IM Ativan, which provides sedation. Haldol is also available in IV form. The use of IV Haldol is generally limited to medical units when the patient is unable to take oral medications and IV access is available.

**V. Antipsychotic Side Effects**

    The following discussion is applicable primarily to the typical antipsychotics. Atypical agents have a relatively low incidence of extrapyramidal effects, tardive dyskinesias, neuroleptic malignant syndrome, and anticholinergic side effects.

    **A. Low-potency agents,** such as chlorpromazine, produce a higher incidence of anticholinergic side effects, sedation and orthostatic hypotension compared to high-potency agents such as haloperidol.

    **B. High-potency agents,** such as haloperidol and fluphenazine, produce a high incidence of extrapyramidal symptoms such as acute dystonic reactions, Parkinsonian syndrome, and akathisia.

    **C. Moderate-potency agents** include trifluoperazine and thiothixene and have side effect profiles in between the low- and high-potency agents.

    **D. Anticholinergic Side Effects**

        **1.** Neuroleptics, especially low-potency agents, such as chlorpromazine and thioridazine, produce anticholinergic side effects such as dry mouth, constipation, blurry vision, and urinary retention.

        **2.** In severe cases, anticholinergic blockade can produce a central anticholinergic syndrome characterized by confusion or delirium, dry flushed skin, dilated pupils and elevated heart rate.

## Classification of Antipsychotic Drugs

| Name | Trade name | Class | Average Dose (mg) | Chlorpromazine Equivalents (mg) | Dopaminergic Effect (D2) | Muscarinic Effect | Alpha-1 Adrenergic Blocking Effect | Antihistamine Effect | Serotonergic Effect |
|---|---|---|---|---|---|---|---|---|---|
| Chlorpromazine | Thorazine | Phenothiazine/Aliphatic | 600-800 | 100 | ++++ | +++ | ++++ | ++++ | ++++ |
| Fluphenazine | Prolixin | Phenothiazine/Piperazine | 10-20 | 2 | ++++ | + | + | ++ | ++ |
| Perphenazine | Trilafon | Phenothiazine/Piperazine | 60-80 | 10 | ++++ | + | ++ | +++ | ++++ |
| Trifluoperazine | Stelazine | Phenothiazine/Piperazine | 30-40 | 5 | ++++ | + | ++ | ++ | +++ |
| Thioridazine | Mellaril | Phenothiazine/Piperidine | 600-800 | 100 | ++++ | ++++ | ++++ | ++++ | ++++ |
| Mesoridazine | Serentil | Phenothiazine/Piperidine | 300-400 | 50 | ++++ | +++ | ++++ | ++++ | +++ |
| Haloperidol | Haldol | Butyrophenone | 10-20 | 2 | ++++ | + | + | + | ++ |
| Clozapine | Clozaril | Dibenzodiazepine | 300-600 | 60 | ++ | ++++ | ++++ | ++++ | ++++ |
| Aripiprazole | Abilify | Quinolone | 15-30 | 2-4 | ++++ | + | ++ | ++ | +++ |
| Loxapine | Loxitane | Dibenzodiazepine | 75-100 | 12.5 | +++ | ++ | +++ | ++++ | ++++ |
| Pimozide | Orap | Diphenylbutylpiperidine | 2-15 | 1 | ++++ | + | + | + | |
| Molindone | Moban | Dihydroindolone | 50-100 | 10 | +++ | ++ | + | + | + |
| Thiothixene | Navane | Thioxanthene | 30-40 | 5 | ++++ | + | ++ | +++ | + |

| Name | Trade name | Class | Average Dose (mg) | Chlorpro-mazine Equivalents (mg) | Dopaminergic Effect (D2) | Muscari-nic Effect | Alpha-1 Adrenergic Blocking Effect | Antihist-amine Effect | Serotoner-gic Effect |
|---|---|---|---|---|---|---|---|---|---|
| Risperidone | Risperdal | Benzisoxazole | 2-8 | 1-2 | ++ | + | +++ | ++ | +++ |
| Olanzapine | Zyprexa Zydis | Thienoben-zodiazepine | 5-20 | 3 | +++ | ++ | ++ | ++ | +++ |
| Quetiapine | Seroquel | Dibenzothiazepine | 400-600 | 50 | + | 0 | ++ | ++ | ++ |
| Ziprasidone | Geodon | Benzisothiazolyl piperzine | 80-160 | 5-10 | +++ | + | + | + | +++ |
| Paliperidone | Invega | Benzisoxazole | 6-12 mg | 2 | ++ | 0 | ++ | ++ | +++ |

**E. Extrapyramidal Side Effects (EPS)**
   1. Neuroleptics, especially the high-potency agents, such as haloperidol, induce involuntary movements known as extrapyramidal side effects. These involuntary movements occur due to blockade of dopamine receptors in the nigrostriatal pathway of the basal ganglia.
   2. **Acute Dystonia**
      a. Acute dystonic reactions are sustained contraction of the muscles of neck (torticollis), eyes (oculogyric crisis), tongue, jaw and other muscle groups, typically occurring within 3-5 days after initiation of the neuroleptic. Dystonias are often very painful and frightening to patients.
      b. Laryngeal spasms can cause airway obstruction, requiring urgent intravenous administration of diphenhydramine.
      c. Dystonic reactions are most frequently induced by high-potency neuroleptics such as haloperidol and fluphenazine (Prolixin), and can occur in young, otherwise healthy persons (particularly younger men) even after a single dose.
      d. Dystonias (other than laryngospasm) should be treated with 1-2 mg of benztropine (Cogentin) IM. The patient may require long-term anticholinergic medication to control the dystonia. Dystonia may resolve over time without changing the dose, but decreasing the dose to the minimum effective dose should be considered if dystonia develops. Dystonias will often improve with a change to a lower potency or atypical agent.
   3. **Drug-Induced Parkinsonian Syndrome**
      a. Patients with Parkinsonian syndrome secondary to neuroleptics present with cogwheel rigidity, mask-like facies, bradykinesia, and shuffling gait. This is similar to patients with idiopathic Parkinson's disease. Onset is usually after 2 weeks. Older patient are at higher risk.
      b. Drug-induced Parkinsonism is treated by adding an anticholinergic agent such as benztropine (Cogentin) or trihexyphenidyl (Artane).
      c. The dopamine releasing agent, amantadine, is also effective.
      d. Parkinsonian symptoms may also improve with a lower dose of neuroleptic or after switching to a low-potency agent such as thioridazine or an atypical agent.
   4. **akathesia**
      a. Akathesia is characterized by strong feelings of inner restlessness, which are manifest by difficulty remaining still and excessive walking or pacing.
      b. Akathesia is very subjectively unpleasant and is associated with medication noncompliance and suicidality.
      c. Akathesia frequently does not improve with anticholinergic medication, but may respond to a beta-blocker such as propranolol in the dose range of 10-40 mg tid or qid. Benzodiazepines such as diazepam are used for refractory cases.
      d. Lowering the medication dose or changing antipsychotic may be required.

**F. Tardive Dyskinesia (TD)**
   1. Tardive dyskinesia is an involuntary movement disorder involving the tongue, mouth, fingers, toes, and other body parts.

2. Tardive dyskinesias are characterized by chewing movements, smacking and licking of the lips, sucking movements, tongue protrusion, blinking, grimaces and spastic facial distortions.
3. All neuroleptics, with the exception of clozapine, produce tardive dyskinesia. The risk of tardive dyskinesia with atypical antipsychotics is substantially decreased compared to typical agents.
4. Antiparkinsonian drugs are of no benefit for tardive dyskinesias and may exacerbate symptoms.
5. When tardive dyskinesia symptoms are observed, the offending drug should be discontinued immediately. Patients who require continued neuroleptic therapy should be switched to an atypical agent or clozapine (if severe).
6. The risk of tardive dyskinesia increases with the duration of neuroleptic exposure, and there is an incidence of 3% per year with typical agents.
7. Most patients have relatively mild cases, but tardive dyskinesia can be debilitating in severe cases. Tardive dyskinesias do not always improve or resolve with discontinuation or lowering of the dose of neuroleptic.

## G. Neuroleptic Malignant Syndrome (NMS)

1. NMS is a rare idiosyncratic reaction, which can be fatal. All neuroleptics, with the exception of clozapine, may produce NMS. The risk of NMS with atypical antipsychotics is substantially decreased.
2. NMS is characterized by severe muscle rigidity, fever, altered mental status, and autonomic instability. Laboratory tests often reveal an elevated WBC, CPK, and liver transaminases.
3. Treatment involves discontinuing the neuroleptic immediately, along with supportive treatment and medications such as amantadine, bromocriptine, and dantrolene. Patients may require treatment in an intensive care unit.

## H. Sedation.
Neuroleptic sedation is related to blockade of H-1 histamine receptors. It is more common with low-potency agents, such as chlorpromazine, compared to high-potency agents, such as haloperidol. Bedtime administration will often reduce daytime sedation.

## I. Weight Gain.
Olanzapine and clozapine are associated with weight gain. Risperidone and quetiapine have relatively less weight liability, while aripiprazole and ziprasidone are considered weight neutral. Blockade of the serotonin 2C and histamine receptors may mediate this effect. Weight gain, especially abdominal or "central adiposity" is associated with increased risk for development of **Metabolic Syndrome** characterized by increased fasting glucose, increased triglycerides, low HDL, and hypertension.

## J. Hyperlipidemia and Diabetes

1. Atypical antipsychotics are associated with elevation of triglycerides and cholesterol and the development of insulin resistance or type II diabetes. Olanzapine and clozapine appear to have the most risk followed by risperidone and quetiapine. Aripiprazole and ziprasidone have little or no risk.
2. Patients with serious mental illness are already at risk for these disorders because of poor diet, unhealthy lifestyle patterns and decreased access to regular medical care; therefore, it is important to aggressively monitor patients for the presence or development of **lipid and glucose dysregulation and encourage adoption of healthy**

lifestyles. The following monitoring schedule of weight, abdominal circumference, and metabolic parameters should be followed (see table below).

| Monitoring Protocol for Patients on Atypical agents (SDAs)* | | | | | | | |
|---|---|---|---|---|---|---|---|
| | Base-line | 4 weeks | 8 weeks | 12 weeks | Quar-terly | An-nu-ally | Every 5 years |
| Per-sonal/-family history | X | | | | | X | |
| Weight (BMI) | X | X | X | X | X | | |
| Blood press-ure | X | | | X | | | |
| Fasting plasma glucose | X | | | X | | | |
| Fasting lipid profile | X | | | X | | | X |
| *More frequent assessments may be warranted based on clinical status | | | | | | | |

K. **Orthostatic Hypotension.** Alpha-1 adrenergic blockade results in orthostatic hypotension which may be serious and can lead to falls and injury. Orthostatic hypotension is especially common with low-potency agents such as chlorpromazine, thioridazine or clozapine. Patients should be advised to get up slowly from recumbent positions.

L. **Cardiac Toxicity.** Cardiac conduction delays can occur with thioridazine, chlorpromazine or pimozide in a dose-related fashion. Ziprasidone may increase the QT interval, but this effect does not appear to be clinically significant. The IM form of ziprasidone does not have this effect on the QT interval. Thioridazine has the greatest effect on QT prolongation and should be used with caution. Ziprasidone should be used with caution in patients with known heart disease, a history of syncope, a family history of sudden death, or a history of congenital prolonged QT interval.

M. **Sexual Side Effects**
   1. Antipsychotics may produce a wide range of sexual dysfunction.
   2. Dopamine receptor (D2) blockade can lead to elevation of prolactin with subsequent gynecomastia, galactorrhea, and menstrual dysfunction.
   3. Retrograde ejaculation, erectile dysfunction, and inhibition of orgasm are also common side effects.

N. **Retinitis Pigmentosa.** Irreversible blindness can rarely occur with a dose of thioridazine greater than 800 mg per day.

O. **Photosensitivity.** Antipsychotic agents often cause photosensitivity and a predisposition to sunburn. Photosensitivity is especially common with low-potency agents, such as chlorpromazine. Blue-purple or gray skin color can also result. This is not always reversible. Patients should be advised to use sunscreen.

P. **Cholestatic jaundice** is a rare hypersensitivity reaction that is most common with chlorpromazine. Cholestatic jaundice is usually reversible after discontinuation of the medication. Most cases develop during the third and fourth weeks of treatment. Treatment should include switching to another class of antipsychotic drug after a drug-free interval.

## VI. Atypical Neuroleptics

A. **Clozapine (Clozaril)** is a dibenzodiazepine derivative and is considered an atypical antipsychotic agent. Clozapine is used for the treatment of patients who have not responded to, or cannot tolerate, other neuroleptics.

   1. Clozapine is associated with a 1% incidence of agranulocytosis, which can be fatal. Weekly monitoring of the WBC is recommended for the first six months of treatment and every two weeks thereafter. When white blood cell counts drop below $3 \times 10^{12}$/liter, clozapine must be discontinued.

   2. Eosinophilia ($>4000$/mm$^3$) may be a precursor of leukopenia. Clozapine should be interrupted until count is below 3000/mm$^3$.

   3. Clozapine is unique in that it does not produce extrapyramidal symptoms, tardive dyskinesia, or NMS. The risk of seizures is increased at dosages above 600 mg per day.

   4. Clozapine causes sedation, orthostatic hypotension, excess salivation (sialorrhea), weight gain, tachycardia, and, rarely, respiratory arrest in conjunction with benzodiazepines. There is no significant elevation of prolactin or subsequent side effects.

B. **Risperidone (Risperdal)**

   1. Risperidone has an atypical side-effect profile with minimal extrapyramidal symptoms at lower doses (up to 4-6 mg). At doses above 6 mg per day, the incidence of EPS increases significantly. The effective dosage range is 2-8 mg/day.

   2. Fatigue and sedation are the most common side effects, followed by weight gain and orthostatic hypotension.

   3. Risperidone can elevate prolactin, leading to gynecomastia, galactorrhea and disruption of the menstrual cycle. Agranulocytosis has not been reported. The incidence of tardive dyskinesia is low.

C. **Olanzapine (Zyprexa)**

   1. Olanzapine has an atypical side-effect profile with a low incidence of extrapyramidal symptoms. The effective dose range is 5-20 mg/day, although some patients may require higher doses. The typical starting dose is 10 mg/day.

   2. Common side effects include sedation, weight gain and dry mouth. Less frequent side effects include orthostatic hypotension, nausea, and tremor. There is no evidence of hemotoxicity. Olanzapine levels may be decreased by tobacco use or carbamazepine. Dose reductions should be made in the elderly.

D. **Quetiapine (Seroquel)**

   1. Quetiapine is an atypical neuroleptic with a very low incidence of EPS. Initial dose is 25-50 mg bid, which is titrated every 1 or 2 days

to a total daily dose of 400-800 mg (given bid or tid) for psychosis. A new XR formulation is available that can be given once a day.

2. Side effects include sedation, orthostatic hypotension and weight gain. Dyspepsia, abdominal pain, and dry mouth may also occur.

3. Initial and periodic eye exams (with slit lamp) are recommended because of the occurrence of cataracts in very high-dose animal studies. Rarely described in humans. Dosage should be reduced in the elderly. Sustained prolactin elevation is not observed.

4. Due to its low-potency and broad therapeutic index, quetiapine has found multiple off-label uses at doses <100mg q day including insomnia, non-specific anxiety,

### E. Ziprasidone (Geodon)

1. Ziprasidone has an atypical side-effect profile with a very low incidence of extrapyramidal symptoms, weight gain, or effects on lipids and glucose. The effective dose range is between 40-80 mg bid.

2. Ziprasidone can increase QT interval. While there are no reports linking this to cardiac arrhythmias, caution should be exercised in patients with pre-existing increased QT interval (from medications or cardiac disease). These patients should have a baseline ECG.

3. Dizziness, nausea, and postural hypotension are the most common side effects. Prolactin elevation can occur.

4. Ziprasidone IM (Geodon IM) is available and can be given 10 mg q 2-4 hours or 20 mg q 4 hours, not to exceed 40 mg/day. Somnolence is more common with the IM form. QT prolongation has not been observed with the IM formulation.

### F. Aripiprazole (Abilify)

1. Aripiprazole has an atypical side-effect profile with a very low incidence of extrapyramidal symptoms. This agent is a dopamine autoreceptor agonist and post-synaptic D2 receptor partial agonist, giving it a unique mechanism of action.

2. Aripiprazole has a low incidence of weight gain, no effect on serum glucose or lipids and no effect on QT interval. Effective dose is 10-30 mg po per day.

3. Side effects occur infrequently but can include akathisia, nausea and tremor.

### G. Paliperidone (Invega)

1. Paliperidone is the active metabolite of risperidone. Patients taking risperidone have significant blood levels of paliperidone. Paliperidone has a similar receptor affinity profile.

2. Paliperidone comes in an extended-release formulation that may improve tolerability as compared to risperidone. It is prescribed in doses from 6-12 mg, once daily.

## VII. Anticholinergic and Antiparkinsonian Agents

A. Anticholinergic and antiparkinsonian agents are used to control the extrapyramidal side effects of antipsychotic agents, including acute dystonic reactions, neuroleptic induced Parkinsonism, and akathisia.

### B. Indications

1. Anticholinergics are drugs of choice for acute dystonias and for drug-induced Parkinsonism. Intramuscular injections of anticholinergic agents are most effective for rapid relief.

2. Anticholinergic agents are less effective for drug-induced akathisia, which often requires addition of a beta-blocker.

3. Antiparkinsonian agents are usually initiated when a patient develops neuroleptic-related extrapyramidal side effects, but they may be given prophylactically in high-risk patients. The anticholinergic agent should be tapered and discontinued after one to six months if possible.

| Classification of Anticholinergic and Antiparkinsonian Agents | | | |
|---|---|---|---|
| **Name** | **Trade Name** | **Class** | **Dose** |
| Benztropine | Cogentin | Anticholinergic | 1-2 mg bid-tid orally or 1-2 mg IM |
| Biperiden | Akineton | Anticholinergic | 2 mg bid-tid orally or 2 mg IM |
| Trihexyphenidyl | Artane | Anticholinergic | 2-5 mg bid-qid |
| Diphenhydramine | Benadryl | Antihistamine/ Anticholinergic | 25-50 mg bid to qid or 25-50 mg IM |
| Amantadine | Symmetrel | Dopamine/ Agonist | 100-150 mg bid |

4. **Side Effects of Anticholinergic Agents**
   a. The most common side effects result from peripheral anticholinergic blockade: dry mouth, constipation, blurry vision, urinary hesitancy, decreased sweating, increased heart rate and ejaculatory dysfunction.
   b. A central anticholinergic syndrome occurs with high doses, or when the agent is combined with other anticholinergic medications. The syndrome is characterized by confusion, dry flushed skin, tachycardia, and pupillary dilation. In severe cases, delirium, hallucinations, arrhythmias, hypotension, seizures and coma may develop.
   c. Anticholinergic drugs are contraindicated in narrow angle glaucoma and should be used cautiously in prostatic hypertrophy or cardiovascular disease.
   d. Amantadine does not have anticholinergic side effects; however, amantadine may cause nausea, insomnia, decreased concentration, dizziness, irritability, anxiety and ataxia. Amantadine is contraindicated in renal failure.

# Antidepressants

I. **Indications for Antidepressant Medication.** Unipolar and bipolar depression, organic mood disorders, anxiety disorders (panic disorder, generalized anxiety disorder, obsessive-compulsive disorder, social phobia), schizoaffective disorder, eating disorder, and impulse control disorders.

II. **Classification of Antidepressants**
   A. **Selective-Serotonin (5HT) Reuptake Inhibitors.** Fluoxetine (Prozac), sertraline (Zoloft), paroxetine (Paxil), fluvoxamine (Luvox), citalopram (Celexa), escitalopram (Lexapro).
   B. **Serotonin/Norepinephrine Reuptake Inhibitors.** Heterocyclics (TCAs), venlafaxine (Effexor), duloxetine (Cymbalta).
   C. **Norepinephrine/Dopamine Reuptake Inhibitors.** Bupropion (Wellbutrin).
   D. **Mixed Serotonin Reuptake Inhibitor/Serotonin Receptor Antagonists.** Trazodone (Desyrel), nefazodone.
   E. **Alpha-2-Adrenergic Antagonist.** Mirtazapine (Remeron).
   F. **Monoamine Oxidase Inhibitors (MAOIs).** Phenelzine, tranylcypromine, isocarboxazid.
   G. **Selective Norepinephrine Reuptake Inhibitor.** Atomoxetine (Strattera) - not FDA approved for depression.

III. **Clinical Use of Antidepressants**
   A. All antidepressants have been shown to have equivalent efficacy. The selection of an agent depends on past history of response, anticipated tolerance to side effects, and coexisting medical problems.
   B. Once a therapeutic dose is reached, symptom improvement typically requires 3-6 weeks. TCAs and bupropion have the narrowest therapeutic index and present the greatest risk in overdose.
   C. If no significant improvement is seen after an adequate trial (4-6 weeks), then the dosage should be increased or one may switch to a medication in another antidepressant class. Alternatively, an augmenting agent such as lithium should be added.
   D. When psychotic symptoms accompany severe cases of depression, concomitant antipsychotic medication is usually required and should be discontinued when the psychosis abates.
   E. Patients with three episodes of major depression should be placed on long-term maintenance treatment.

IV. **Side Effects**
   A. **Cardiac Toxicity**
      1. Tricyclic antidepressants may slow cardiac conduction, resulting in intraventricular conduction delay, prolongation of the QT interval, and AV block. Patients with preexisting conduction problems are predisposed to arrhythmias; therefore, TCAs should not be used in patients with conduction defects, arrhythmias, or a history of a recent MI.
      2. SSRIs, venlafaxine, bupropion, mirtazapine, and nefazodone have no effects on cardiac conduction.
   B. **Anticholinergic Adverse Drug Reactions.** Dry mouth, blurred vision, constipation, and urinary retention.
   C. **Antihistaminergic Adverse Drug Reactions.** Sedation, weight gain.
   D. **Adverse Drug Reactions Caused by Alpha-1 Blockade.** Orthostatic hypotension, sedation, sexual dysfunction.
   E. **Serotonergic Activation.** GI symptoms (nausea, diarrhea), insomnia or somnolence, agitation, tremor, anorexia, headache, and sexual dysfunction can occur with SSRIs, especially early in treatment.
   F. Bupropion, mirtazapine and nefazodone are the least likely to produce sexual side effects.
   G. **Discontinuation Syndrome.** Sudden cessation of SSRIs is associated with typical symptoms of dizziness, fatigue, headache, nausea, insomnia,

shock-like sensations. While not dangerous, the discontinuation syndrome is unpleasant and can be avoided by taper of SSRIs. Intensity of the syndrome is related to half-life with short half-life SSRIs being associated with more rapid onset, more intense but short-lived symptoms. Cross-titration is not necessary when switching from one SSRI to another with the exception of paroxetine. Sudden cessation of paroxetine will provoke SSRI discontinuation syndrome and a cholinergic rebound syndrome (nausea, vomiting, diarrhea, sialorrhea, diaphoresis) even if the patient begins another SSRI immediately.

**H. MAOIs.** The most common adverse drug reaction is hypotension. Patients are also at risk for hypertensive crisis if foods high in tyramine content or sympathomimetic drugs are consumed. Despite the infrequent use of MAOIs, they remain important for the treatment of refractory depression.

## Commonly Used Antidepressants

| Drug | Recommended dosage | Comments |
| --- | --- | --- |
| **Secondary Amine Tricyclics** | | |
| **Class as a whole:** Side effects include anticholinergic effects (dry mouth, blurred vision, constipation) and alpha-blocking effects (sedation, orthostatic hypotension, cardiac rhythm disturbances). May lower seizure threshold. | | |
| Desipramine (Norpramin, generics) | Initial dosage 25-50 mg qhs, average dose 150-250 mg/d, May require dose of 300 mg/d. [10, 25, 50, 75, 100, 150 mg] | May have CNS stimulant effect. |
| Protriptyline (Vivactil) | Initial dose of 5 mg q am increasing to 15-40 mg/d in bid dosing [5, 10 mg] | Less sedating than other TCAs. |
| Nortriptyline (Pamelor) | Initial dose 25 mg qhs, increasing to 75-150 mg/d; monitor levels to achieve serum level between 50-150 ng/mL. [10, 25, 50, 75 mg] | Sedating. Serum levels available. |

| Drug | Recommended dosage | Comments |
|---|---|---|
| **Tertiary Amine Tricyclics** | | |
| **Class as a whole:** Anticholinergic effects and orthostatic hypotension may be more severe than with secondary amine tricyclics. All are contraindicated in glaucoma and should be used with caution in urinary retention and cardiovascular disorders. | | |
| Amitriptyline (Elavil, generics) | Initial dose of 25-50 mg qhs increasing to 150-250 mg/d. May be given as single hs dose. [10, 25, 50, 75, 100, 150 mg] | High sedation. High anticholinergic activity. |
| Clomipramine (Anafranil) | Initial dose of 25-50 mg qhs increasing to 150-250 mg/d; may be given once qhs [25, 50, 75 mg] | Relatively high sedation, anticholinergic activity, and seizure risk. |
| Doxepin (Sinequan, Adapin) | Initial dose of 25-50 mg/d, increasing to 150-300 mg/d. [10, 25, 50, 75, 100, 150 mg] | High sedation, often used as a hypnotic at a dosage of 25-150 mg qhs. |
| Imipramine (Tofranil, generics) | 75 mg/d in a single dose qhs, increasing to 150 mg/d; max 300 mg/d. [10, 25, 50 mg] | Relatively high sedation. Also used to treat enuresis. |
| **Tetracyclic** | | |
| Mirtazapine (Remeron) | 15 mg qhs initially increasing to 30-45 mg qhs over days to weeks [15, 30 mg] | Sedation and appetite stimulation inversely proportional to dose. Minimal effect on hepatic enzymes. |
| Maprotiline (Ludiomil, generics) | 75 mg qhs initially, Usual effective dose 150 mg/d, max 225 mg/d. [25, 50, 75 mg] | Sedating. Substantial risk of seizures; maculopapular rash in 3-10%. Rarely used. |
| Amoxapine (Asendin) | Initial dosage 25-50 mg qhs, increase to 200-300 mg/d if necessary. Max 600 mg/d. [25, 50, 100, 150 mg] | May be associated with tardive dyskinesia, neuroleptic malignant syndrome, galactorrhea. Rarely used. |
| **Selective-Serotonin Reuptake Inhibitors (SSRIs)** | | |
| **Class as a whole:** Common side effects include sexual dysfunction, headache, nausea, anxiety, mild sedation, insomnia, anorexia. | | |
| Fluoxetine (Prozac) | 10-20 mg/d initially, taken in AM; may require up to 80 mg/day for OCD and bulimia [10, 20 mg capsules / 20 mg/5 mL soln, 90 mg weekly tablet] | May be activating. Longest half-life of any antidepressant (2-9 days). Discontinue 2 months before pregnancy. Significant inhibition of CYP2D6 |

| Drug | Recommended dosage | Comments |
|------|-------------------|----------|
| Fluvoxamine (Luvox) | 50 mg hs initially, then increase up to 300 mg/day [25,50, 100 mg] | Moderate sedation. Significant inhibition of CYP1A2 |
| Paroxetine (Paxil, Paxil CR [extended release]) | 20 mg hs initially; max of 80 mg/d. Elderly starting dosage, 10 mg/d [10, 20, 30, 40 mg; 10 mg/5mL oral solution; 12.5, 25, 37.5mg continuous release formulation] | Moderate sedation and dry mouth. Significant inhibition of CYP2D6. |
| Citalopram (Celexa) | 20-60 mg/d [10, 20, 40 mg tabs; 10mg/5mL oral solution] | Minimal sedation, activation, or inhibition of hepatic enzymes. |
| Escitalopram (Lexapro) | 10-20 mg qd [5, 10, 20 mg tabs; 5mg/5mL oral solution] | Minimal sedation, activation, or inhibition of hepatic enzymes. |
| Sertraline (Zoloft) | 50 qd, increasing as needed to max of 200 mg/d [25,50, 100 mg tabs; 20mg/mL oral suspension] | Minimal sedation, activation, or inhibition of hepatic enzymes. |
| **Miscellaneous** | | |
| Duloxetine (Cymbalta) | 20 mg bid increasing as needed to an average of 30 mg bid and maximum of 60 mg bid. [20, 30, and 60 mg capsules] | Nausea, decreased appetite, dry mouth, dizziness, and sexual dysfunction. Helpful for syndromes associated with depression. Effective for diabetic neuropathy. |
| Nefazodone | 50-100 mg bid initially, increasing to 150-300 mg bid. [50,100, 150, 200, 250 mg] | Headache, dry mouth, blurred vision somnolence, postural hypotension, minimal sexual side effects or inhibition of hepatic enzymes. Rare reports of liver failure. |

| Drug | Recommended dosage | Comments |
|------|-------------------|----------|
| Venlafaxine (Effexor, Effexor XR) | 37.5 mg bid initially increasing to 150-225 mg/day in divided dose. Extended release (XR): 37.5-75 mg/day increasing to 150-225 mg/day [25, 37.5, 50, 75, 100 mg] [XR: 37.5, 75, 100] | Mild hypertension possible. Common side effects: Nausea, somnolence, insomnia, dizziness, sexual dysfunction, headache, dry mouth, anxiety. Minimal or no inhibition of hepatic enzymes. |
| Bupropion (Wellbutrin, Wellbutrin SR, Wellbutrin XL, Zyban) | 100 mg bid initially increasing to 100 mg tid over 5 days. Slow release (SR): begin with 100-150 mg qd for 3 days, increasing to 150 mg bid over 4-7 days [75, 100 mg] [SR: 100, 150, 200 mg] [XL: 150, 300 mg tabs] | Agitation, dry mouth, insomnia, headache, nausea, vomiting, constipation, tremor. Good choice if sexual side effects from other agents. Significant inhibition of CYP2D6. |
| Trazodone (Desyrel) | 50-100 mg qhs initially increasing gradually to dose of 300-600 mg/day [50, 100, 150, 300 mg] | Rare association with priapism. Orthostatic hypotension. Highly sedating. |

# Mood Stabilizers

## I. Indications for Mood Stabilizers

**A.** Mood stabilizers are the drugs of choice for bipolar disorder, schizoaffective disorder, and cyclothymia. They are effective for acute mania and for prophylaxis of mania and depression in bipolar disorders. Mood stabilizers are less effective for bipolar depression.

**B.** These agents are sometimes effective for impulse control disorders and aggressive behavior.

## II. Valproic Acid (Depakote)

**A.** Valproic acid has become the mood stabilizer of choice due to its favorable side-effect profile and lower toxicity in overdose compared to lithium or carbamazepine.

**B.** Valproic acid is effective for bipolar disorder, schizoaffective disorder, and cyclothymia. It is also used for impulse control disorders and aggression in Cluster B personality disorders, dementia, or mental retardation.

**C.** Valproic acid is more effective in rapid cycling and mixed state episode bipolar disorder than lithium.

**D. Treatment Guidelines**

1. Valproate usually requires two weeks to take full effect, but a trial of four to six weeks should be completed before evaluating efficacy.

2. Serum levels, CBC, platelet count, and PT/PTT should be obtained weekly during the first month of treatment. Steady state levels can be measured in 2-3 days.

3. Divalproex (Depakote) is the best tolerated form of valproate. Divalproex is initiated at a dosage of 20 µg/kg for rapid stabilization of mania. This roughly corresponds to 500 mg tid or 750 bid with titration up to a serum level of 50-125 mg/mL. The average dose is between

1500-3000 mg/day. Depakote ER (extended release) tablets (500 mg) allow for once-a-day dosing. Depakote ER has 80-90% bioavailability compared to Depakote.

4. Elderly patients require doses of approximately half that of younger adults.

5. Valproate is more benign in overdose than lithium or carbamazepine.

## III. Lithium (Eskalith, Eskalith CR, Lithonate)

A. Lithium, in addition to being an antimanic agent, possesses modest but significant antidepressant properties. However, lithium is less effective than valproate (Depakote) in rapid cycling mania.

B. Regular and slow-release forms of lithium carbonate are available and either form may be given twice daily initially switching to once-daily dosing after several weeks.

C. Healthy young adults can usually tolerate 300-600 mg of lithium carbonate, twice daily at the start of therapy. The dose is increased over seven to ten days until the plasma level is 0.80-1.20 mEq/L (0.80 to 1.20 mMol/L). Serum lithium levels are measured 12 hours after the preceding dose of lithium.

D. **Common side effects of lithium** include polyuria, thirst, edema, weight gain, fine tremor, mild nausea (especially if the drug is not taken with food), and diarrhea.

E. **Lithium toxicity** is manifested by coarse tremor, stupor, ataxia, seizures, persistent headache, vomiting, slurred speech, confusion, incontinence, and arrhythmias. Toxicity may occur when a patient becomes ill and ceases to eat and drink normally, but continues to take lithium. A patient who cannot eat and drink normally should temporarily discontinue lithium.

F. Serum lithium levels >2.0 (trough) can produce permanent neurological impairment.

G. Nonsteroidal anti-inflammatory drugs, such as ibuprofen or aspirin, and ACE inhibitors, elevate the plasma lithium level. Lithium levels should be carefully monitored. A reduction of lithium dose may be required.

H. Lithium levels rise 20-25 percent when diuretics, such as chlorothiazide (Diuril), are initiated. A reduction of lithium dose may be required.

I. Laboratory evaluation prior to beginning treatment with lithium should include blood urea nitrogen, creatinine, electrolytes, fasting blood sugar, TSH, free T4 levels, and an ECG in patients over 40 years or with pre-existing cardiac disease.

J. Side effects, such as tremor, may be reduced by using divided doses or slow-release formulations. The usual adult dosage ranges from 600-2400 mg/day. Two weeks are required for effect, and the drug should be continued for four to eight weeks before evaluating efficacy.

K. Serum levels must be drawn weekly for the first one to two months, then every two to four weeks. Serum levels should be kept between 0.8-1.2 mMol/L

L. Serum creatinine and TSH are monitored every 6 months.

M. Side Effects

1. **Gastrointestinal distress** (diarrhea, nausea) may be reduced by giving the medication with meals or by switching to a sustained release preparation.

2. **Tremor** is most common in the hands. Tremor is treated by lowering the dosage or by adding low-dose propranolol (10-40 mg tid-qid).

3. **Diabetes insipidus** may result from lithium administration. It presents with polyuria and polydipsia. Treatment consists of amiloride

administration, in doses of 5-20 mg per day with frequent monitoring of lithium and potassium levels.

4. **Hypothyroidism** may result from lithium and is treated with levothyroxine.

5. **Dermatological** side effects include acne, which can be controlled with benzoyl peroxide or topical antibiotics. Lithium can induce or exacerbate psoriasis, which usually responds to discontinuation of lithium.

6. **Elevated WBC** count, usually between 11-15 thousand, is frequently observed and requires no treatment.

7. **Cardiac** side effects include T-wave flattening or inversion and rare arrhythmias, which require discontinuation of lithium.

8. **Lithium toxicity** may occur when levels exceed 1.5 mEq/liter. Toxicity presents with emesis, diarrhea, confusion, ataxia, and cardiac arrhythmias. Seizures, coma and death may occur at levels above 2.5 mEq/liter. Treatment of overdose may require hemodialysis.

## IV. Carbamazepine (Tegretol)

### A.
Carbamazepine is used in patients who do not respond to lithium. Carbamazepine is dosed bid or tid to minimize side effects.

### B. Treatment Guidelines

1. **Pretreatment Evaluations.** CBC with differential and platelets, liver function tests, EKG, electrolytes, creatinine and physical examination.

2. Carbamazepine requires two weeks to take effect, but a therapeutic trial should last at least four to eight weeks.

3. Obtain serum levels (target is 8-12 µg/mL) along with a CBC, liver function tests and electrolytes weekly for a month. The WBC should be monitored more frequently if the white count begins to drop.

4. After the first month, levels may be drawn less frequently.

5. Carbamazepine induces its own metabolism and carbamazepine levels will decline between three and eight weeks. At this time, the dosage may need to be increased to maintain a therapeutic blood level of 8-12 µg/mL.

### C. Side Effects

1. The most serious side effects of carbamazepine are agranulocytosis and aplastic anemia, which occur at a frequency of 1 in 20,000.

2. Carbamazepine should be discontinued if the total WBC count drops below 3,000 cells/mcL, or if the absolute neutrophil count drops below 1,500 cells/mcL, or if the platelet count drops below 100,000 cells/mcL.

3. Hepatitis may rarely occur, which may require discontinuation of carbamazepine. Mild elevations in liver function tests are seen in most patients and this does not require discontinuation of the drug.

4. Stevens-Johnson syndrome, a severe dermatologic condition, is a rare side effect of carbamazepine and requires immediate discontinuation of therapy. Stevens-Johnson syndrome begins with widespread purpuric macules, leading to epidermolysis necrosis with erosion of mucus membranes, epidermis and severe constitutional symptoms.

5. Carbamazepine may also cause ataxia, confusion, and tremors (usually with high doses or toxicity). If this occurs the carbamazepine dose should be decreased to achieve serum levels of 8-12 µg/mL.

6. Carbamazepine decreases serum levels of acetaminophen, antipsychotics, benzodiazepines, oral contraceptives, corticosteroids, cyclosporine, doxycycline, phenytoin, methadone, theophylline, thyroid

supplements, valproate, warfarin, and ethosuximide. Serum levels are decreased by clomipramine and phenytoin.

   **7.** Carbamazepine is more benign in overdose than lithium.

**D. Side Effects**

   **1.** Gastrointestinal distress (nausea and vomiting) is the most common side effect, and these symptoms often improve with coadministration with food.

   **2.** Sedation is common and usually abates in the first few weeks. Hepatitis and pancreatitis are rare complications and usually occur during the first several months.

   **3.** Mild elevations of liver function occur in many patients and require no special treatment except frequent monitoring of liver enzymes. Thrombocytopenia is rare and may require discontinuation of the drug if levels drop below 100,000.

   **4.** Elevation of serum ammonia is a rare complication and is often benign. Elevated ammonia may, however, be an indicator of severe hepatotoxicity, especially if accompanied by confusion.

**V. Gabapentin (Neurontin)**

  **A.** Controlled studies do not currently support the efficacy of gabapentin in cyclical mood disorders.

  **B.** Gabapentin has been used primarily as an adjunctive treatment to other mood stabilizers and/or antidepressants. It may be helpful for anxiety, irritability and assist with sleep.

  **C. Treatment Guidelines**

   **1.** Renal function should be evaluated before initiating treatment because gabapentin is excreted unchanged renally. Impaired renal function is not a contraindication to gabapentin; however, the dosage should be reduced in patients with impaired renal function.

   **2.** Starting dose is 300 mg q day with titration up to an average daily dose of 900-1800 mg q day in divided doses. Some studies have used up to 3600 mg/day. Given its short half-life, the time between doses should not exceed 12 hours. Serum levels are not useful because no therapeutic window has been established.

   **3.** Therapeutic effects can be seen in 2-4 weeks.

  **D. Side Effects**

   **1.** The most common side effects are somnolence, fatigue, ataxia, nausea and vomiting and dizziness. Gabapentin has been reported to rarely cause anxiety, irritability, agitation and depression.

   **2.** Weight gain is an occasional side effect of gabapentin.

**VI. Lamotrigine (Lamictal)**

  **A.** Lamotrigine is an anticonvulsant. It is indicated for the treatment of bipolar depression. It also appears to be more effective in the treatment of depression compared to other mood stabilizers, prompting some clinicians to use it in the treatment of resistant unipolar depression.

  **B.** Lamotrigine has been successful as monotherapy and as adjunctive treatment to other mood stabilizers and/or antidepressants.

  **C. Treatment Guidelines**

   **1.** Pre-treatment evaluation should include an assessment of renal and hepatic function because both are involved in its excretion.

   **2.** The initial dosage is 25 mg qd, increased weekly to 50 mg/day, 100 mg/day, then 200 mg/day. Up to 400 mg may be required to treat depression. Dosing can be either once or twice a day.

3. Serum levels are not useful because the therapeutic window has not been determined.
4. Coadministration with other anticonvulsants can affect serum levels and should be used with caution.
5. Therapeutic effect may be seen in 2-4 weeks.

**D. Side Effects**
1. The most common side effects are dizziness, sedation, headache, diplopia, ataxia or decreased coordination. The side effect most likely to cause discontinuation of the drug is rash (10%), which can be quite severe. Rash is most common when lamotrigine is initiated at higher doses or when titration is rapid.
2. The incidence of serious rash in adults is 0.3% and can include Stevens-Johnson syndrome. The risk for serious rash is higher in children (0.8%).
3. Lamotrigine has been reported to cause irritability, agitation, anxiety, mania and depression.
4. Carbamazepine will lower lamotrigine levels and valproate will increase lamotrigine levels.

**VII. Topiramate (Topamax)**
**A.** Topiramate is an anticonvulsant that has failed clinical trials as a treatment for mania. Despite this lack of efficacy data, it continues to be used as an adjunctive treatment in bipolar disorder.

**B. Treatment Guidelines**
1. The starting dose is 25-50 mg/day, increasing at increments of 25-50 mg per week to a target dose of 200-400 mg/day, given in single dose or bid. Therapeutic effects are seen in 2-4 weeks.
2. Topiramate is primarily excreted unchanged in urine and has no effect on liver enzymes. Plasma levels of topiramate can be reduced up to 50% when combined with carbamazepine and to a lesser degree with valproate. Topiramate can reduce clearance of phenytoin and impair the efficacy of oral contraceptives.

**C. Side Effects**
1. The most common side effects are sedation, dizziness, ataxia, vision problems, speech problems, memory impairment, and problems with language processing.
2. Unlike other mood stabilizers, topiramate does not cause weight gain and may promote weight loss.

**VIII. Tiagabine (Gabitril)**
**A.** Tiagabine is a new anticonvulsant that is being studied for efficacy as a mood stabilizer. Uncontrolled studies suggest that it may be useful as an adjunct to other mood stabilizers. Tiagabine may have some efficacy for chronic pain and anxiety.
**B.** Tiagabine is hepatically metabolized, but it does not appear to induce hepatic enzymes. Tiagabine does not affect the metabolism of other medications. Clearance may be decreased up to 60% when combined with carbamazepine, phenytoin, or phenobarbital.
**C.** The initial dose is 4 mg/day, increasing by 4 mg at weekly intervals to 12 mg/day, given in single dose or bid. The typical maintenance dose for seizures is 24-32 mg/day given bid or qid.
**D.** The most common side effects are dizziness, lack of energy, somnolence, nausea, nervousness, and tremor.

### IX. Oxcarbazepine (Trileptal)

**A.** Oxcarbazepine is a new anticonvulsant that is being studied for efficacy as a mood stabilizer. Controlled studies suggest that it is effective in mania at doses between 900-2400 mg/day.

**B.** The most common side effects are somnolence, dizziness, diplopia, ataxia, nausea, vomiting and rash.

### X. Levetiracetam (Keppra) has been approved for treatment of partial seizures. Its efficacy for affective illness is unknown.

## Mood Stabilizers

| Name | Trade Name | Dosage Forms | Dose Range | Therapeutic Drug Levels |
|------|-----------|-------------|-----------|------------------------|
| Divalproex sodium | Depakote | 125, 250 or 500 mg; 125 mg sprinkle capsules | 500-4000 mg in bid dosing | 50-125 mcg/mL |
| Divalproex sodium extended release | Depakote ER | 250 or 500 mg | 500-4000 mg in bid dosing | 50-125 mcg/mL |
| Lithium carbonate | Lithonate, Eskalith | 300 mg | 600-2400 mg | 0.8-1.2 mEq/liter |
| Lithium carbonate, slow release | Lithobid, Eskalith CR | 300 or 450 mg | 600-2400 mg | 0.8-1.2 mEq/liter |
| Lithium citrate | Cibalith-S | 8 mEq/5 mL | 10-40 mL | 0.8-1.2 mEq/liter |
| Carbamaze-pine | Tegretol, generics | 100 or 200 mg | 400-1800 mg in bid-qid dosing | 8-12 mcg/mL |
| | | Liquid: 100 mg/5 mL | 400-1800 mg in bid- qid dosing | 8-12 mcg/mL |
| Valproic acid | Depakene | 250 mg | 500-3000 mg in bid dosing | 50-125 mcg/mL |
| Gabapentin | Neurontin | 100, 300, 400 mg | 300-800 mg tid | not applicable |
| Lamotrigine | Lamictal | 25, 100, 150, 200 mg | 100-400 mg | not applicable |
| Tiagabine | Gabitril | 4, 12, 16, 20 mg | 12-mg qd or in divided dose | not applicable |
| Topiramate | Topamax | 25, 100, 200 mg | 200-400 mg qd or in divided dose | not applicable |

# Antianxiety Agents

## I. Benzodiazepines

**A. Indications.** Benzodiazepines are used for the treatment of anxiety disorders, insomnia, seizure disorders, and alcohol detoxification. They are also effective adjunctive agents for agitated psychotic or depressive states.

1. The primary indications for long-term treatment are chronic anxiety disorders such as generalized anxiety disorder and panic disorder. All benzodiazepines induce tolerance and are addictive. Short courses of treatment should be used whenever possible. When benzodiazepines are discontinued, the drug should be tapered slowly. Long-acting agents, such as clonazepam and diazepam, are preferable for long-term treatment because they cause less withdrawal and require less frequent dosing.

2. The 3-hydroxy-benzodiazepines (lorazepam, alprazolam, oxazepam) have no active metabolites and are the agents of choice in patients with impaired liver function.

3. Acute agitation usually is treated with lorazepam (Ativan), 2 mg IM because it is well tolerated and effective in most patients.

**B. Side Effects**

1. **Sedation** is the most common and universal side effect of benzodiazepines. Tolerance to sedative effects often occurs during the first few weeks of treatment.

2. **Cognitive Dysfunction.** Anterograde amnesia is common after benzodiazepine use, especially with high-potency agents (alprazolam) or short-acting agents (triazolam).

3. **Miscellaneous Side Effects**

   a. Benzodiazepines may produce ataxia, slurred speech, and dizziness. Respiratory depression can occur at high doses, especially in combination with alcohol or respiratory disorders, such as chronic obstructive pulmonary disease.

   b. Benzodiazepines are contraindicated in pregnancy or lactation.

| Antianxiety Agents | | | | |
|---|---|---|---|---|
| Name | Trade Name | Dose (mg) | Dose Equivalence | Half-Life of Metabolites (hours) |
| Alprazolam | Xanax | 0.25-2 tid/qid | 0.5 | 6-20 |
| Chlordiazepoxide | Librium | 25-50 tid/qid | 10 | 30-100 |
| Clonazepam | Klonopin | 0.25-2 bid/tid | 0.25 | 18-50 |
| Clorazepate | Tranxene | 7.5 -30 bid | 7.5 | 30-100 |
| Diazepam | Valium | 2-15 bid/tid | 5 | 30-100 |

| Name | Trade Name | Dose (mg) | Dose Equivalence | Half-Life of Metabolites (hours) |
|------|-----------|-----------|------------------|----------------------------------|
| Halazepam | Paxipam | 20-80 bid | 20 | 30-100 |
| Lorazepam | Ativan | 0.5–2 tid/qid | 1 | 10-20 |
| Oxazepam | Serax | 15-30 tid/qid | 15 | 8-12 |

## II. Buspirone (BuSpar)

**A.** Buspirone is a nonbenzodiazepine anxiolytic agent of the azaperone class.

**B. Indications**

1. Buspirone (BuSpar) is indicated for anxiety disorders, such as generalized anxiety disorder but not panic disorder.
2. Buspirone may also be an effective adjunctive agent in the treatment resistant depression. Buspirone may be added in a dosage of 15-60 mg/day if a patient has had a suboptimal response to a 3-6 week trial of an antidepressant.

**C. Dosage**

1. The starting dose is 5 mg two to three times a day. Gradually increase to a maximum dosage of 60 mg per day over several weeks. Many patients respond to a total dose of 30-40 mg per day in two to three divided doses.
2. At least two weeks are required before clinical improvement occurs.

**D. Side Effects**

1. Buspirone is generally well tolerated; the most common side effects are nausea, headaches, dizziness, and insomnia.
2. Buspirone is not addicting and has no withdrawal syndrome or tolerance. It does not produce sedation or potentiate the effects of alcohol.

### References
References, see page 120.

# *Somatic Therapies*

## Electroconvulsive Therapy

Electroconvulsive therapy (ECT) is a highly effective treatment for depression, with a response rate of 90%, compared to a 70% response rate for antidepressants.

### I. Indications
   A. Electroconvulsive therapy is effective for major depressive disorder, bipolar affective disorder (to treat mania and depression), catatonic stupor, and acute psychosis.
   B. Electroconvulsive therapy could be used as a first-line treatment for depression, but this rarely occurs. It is considered early in the treatment course if the pt is catatonic, actively attempting to harm themselves, unable to tolerate antidepressants for medical reasons or is refusing to eat/drink as a result of depression.
   C. Special populations in which ECT is highly effective include: elderly patients (especially those who cannot tolerate therapeutic doses of antidepressants), pregnant women (reported safe in all 3 trimesters and even post-partum) and treatment-resistant patients.
   D. Depression in Parkinson's disease responds to ECT with the added benefit of improvement of the movement disorder.

### II. Electroconvulsive Therapy Evaluation
   A. Pretreatment evaluation should include a complete a history and physical, routine laboratory tests (CBC, electrolytes, liver enzymes, urinalysis, thyroid function), EKG, chest X-ray, spinal X-ray series, and brain CT scan.
   B. Informed consent should be obtained 24 hours prior to the first treatment. A second psychiatrist, not involved in the treatment of the patient, must also examine the patient and document the appropriateness of ECT and the patient's ability to give informed consent.
   C. **Electroconvulsive Therapy Procedure**
      1. The patient should be NPO for at least eight hours and blood pressure, cardiac activity, oxygen content, and the electroencephalogram should be monitored.
      2. A short-acting barbiturate, such as methohexital, is administered for anesthesia. A tourniquet (to prevent paralysis) is applied to one extremity in order to monitor the motor component of the seizure.
      3. Muscle paralysis is then induced by succinylcholine. After an airway has been established, a rubber mouth block is then placed and an electrical stimulus is applied to induce the seizure.
      4. The duration of the seizure is monitored by EEG and by observing the isolated extremity.
   D. **Dose**
      1. The seizure must last a minimum of 25 seconds and should not last longer than two minutes. If the seizure lasts less than 25 seconds, wait one minute and then stimulate again. Electrical stimulation should be discontinued after three failed attempts.

2. If seizures exceed two minutes, intravenous diazepam is used to terminate the seizure.
3. Treatments are given two to three times per week. A minimum of six treatments are usually required (common course is 8-12 treatments). The first three are often performed with bilateral electrode placement. Up to twenty treatments may be necessary before maximum response is attained.

III. **Contraindications to Electroconvulsive Therapy** include intracranial mass, recent stroke and recent MI. The procedure is very safe, and the complication rate is comparable to that of anesthesia alone.

IV. **Side Effects of Electroconvulsive Therapy**
   A. **Memory Loss.** Retrograde and anterograde amnesia of the events surrounding the treatment is common. Loss of recent memory usually resolves within a few days to a few weeks. A small number of patients complain of persistent memory difficulties after several months.
   B. Headache is common after ECT, and it usually resolves with analgesics in a few hours.

V. **Maintenance Electroconvulsive Therapy**
   A. Infrequently, maintenance ECT may be required for up to six months after the end of the initial series of 8-12 treatments.
   B. Treatments are given weekly for one month and then gradually tapered to one treatment every four to five weeks. Some patients may require long-term treatment.

# Transcranial Magnetic Stimulation

I. **Mechanism**
   A. **Repetitive transcranial magnetic stimulation (rTMS)** uses an electric coil to generate magnetic fields that stimulate the cerebral cortex. It is very well tolerated by patients and, in contrast to ECT, does not require the use of anesthesia and does not appear to cause cognitive impairment.
   B. Randomized, controlled studies of rTMS have produced conflicting results. A systematic review concluded that there is no strong evidence of benefit with rTMS in depressed patients. A subsequent randomized trial of rTMS in 60 patients with treatment-resistant depression showed a significantly higher rate of response in two active treatment groups compared with placebo; the absolute benefit, however, was relatively small.

II. **Adverse effects** are limited to mild pain or discomfort at the stimulation site and possible facial twitching. TMS has not been approved by the FDA for the treatment of depression.

# Vagus Nerve Stimulation

Vagus nerve stimulation (VNS) was originally developed and approved for the treatment of refractory seizure disorders. VNS appears to be effective in the treatment of moderate treatment-resistant depression. A pacemaker-like pulse generator is implanted under the skin in the upper left chest. A stimulation electrode connected to the generator is tunneled from the chest to the neck where it is attached to the left vagus nerve. The most common adverse effect associated with VNS is voice alteration or hoarseness.

**References**

American Psychiatric Association. Diagnostic and Statistical Manual of Mental Disorders. 4th edition, Washington, D.C., American Psychiatric Association, 1994.

Additional references may be obtained at www.ccspublishing.com/ccs

# Selected DSM-IV Codes

## ATTENTION-DEFICIT AND DISRUPTIVE BEHAVIOR DISORDERS

| | |
|---|---|
| 314.xx | Attention-Deficit/Hyperactivity Disorder |
| .01 | Combined Type |
| .00 | Predominantly Inattentive Type |
| .01 | Predominantly Hyperactive-Impulsive Type |

## DEMENTIA

| | |
|---|---|
| 290.xx | Dementia of the Alzheimer's Type, With Early Onset *(also code 331.0 Alzheimer's disease on Axis III)* |
| .10 | Uncomplicated |
| 290.xx | Dementia of the Alzheimer's Type, With Late Onset *(also code 331.0 Alzheimer's disease on Axis III)* |
| .0 | Uncomplicated |
| 290.xx | Vascular Dementia |
| .40 | Uncomplicated |

## MENTAL DISORDERS DUE TO A GENERAL MEDICAL CONDITION NOT ELSEWHERE CLASSIFIED

| | |
|---|---|
| 310.1 | Personality Change Due to... *[Indicate the General Medical Condition]* |

## ALCOHOL-RELATED DISORDERS

| | |
|---|---|
| 303.90 | Alcohol Dependence |
| 305.00 | Alcohol Abuse |
| 291.8 | Alcohol-Induced Mood Disorder |
| 291.8 | Alcohol-Induced Anxiety Disorder |

## AMPHETAMINE (OR AMPHETAMINE-LIKE)-RELATED DISORDERS

| | |
|---|---|
| 304.40 | Amphetamine Dependence |
| 305.70 | Amphetamine Abuse |

## COCAINE-RELATED DISORDERS

| | |
|---|---|
| 304.20 | Cocaine Dependence |
| 305.60 | Cocaine Abuse |

## OPIOID-RELATED DISORDERS

| | |
|---|---|
| 304.00 | Opioid Dependence |
| 305.50 | Opioid Abuse |

## SEDATIVE-, HYPNOTIC-, OR ANXIOLYTIC-RELATED DISORDERS

| | |
|---|---|
| 304.10 | Sedative, Hypnotic, or Anxiolytic Dependence |
| 305.40 | Sedative, Hypnotic, or Anxiolytic Abuse |

## POLYSUBSTANCE-RELATED DISORDER

| | |
|---|---|
| 304.80 | Polysubstance Dependence |

## SCHIZOPHRENIA AND OTHER PSYCHIATRIC DISORDERS

| | |
|---|---|
| 295.xx | Schizophrenia |
| .30 | Paranoid Type |
| .10 | Disorganized Type |
| .20 | Catatonic Type |
| .90 | Undifferentiated Type |
| .60 | Residual Type |
| 295.40 | Schizophreniform Disorder |
| 295.70 | Schizoaffective Disorder |
| 297.1 | Delusional Disorder |
| 298.8 | Brief Psychotic Disorder |
| 297.3 | Shared Psychotic Disorder |
| 293.xx | Psychotic Disorder Due to... |
| .81 | With Delusions |
| .82 | With Hallucinations |
| 298.9 | Psychotic Disorder NOS |

## DEPRESSIVE DISORDERS

| | |
|---|---|
| 296.xx | Major Depressive Disorder |
| .2x | Single Episode |
| .3x | Recurrent |
| 300.4 | Dysthymic Disorder |
| 311 | Depressive Disorder NOS |

## BIPOLAR DISORDERS

| | |
|---|---|
| 296.xx | Bipolar I Disorder, |
| .0x | Single Manic Episode |
| .40 | Most Recent Episode Hypomanic |
| .4x | Most Recent Episode Manic |
| .6x | Most Recent Episode Mixed |
| .5x | Most Recent Episode Depressed |
| .7 | Most Recent Episode Unspecified |
| 296.89 | Bipolar II Disorder |
| 301.13 | Cyclothymic Disorder |
| 296.80 | Bipolar Disorder NOS |
| 293.83 | Mood Disorder Due to... *[Indicate the General Medical Condition]* |

## ANXIETY DISORDERS

| | |
|---|---|
| 300.01 | Panic Disorder Without Agoraphobia |
| 300.21 | Panic Disorder With Agoraphobia |
| 300.22 | Agoraphobia Without History of Panic Disorder |
| 300.29 | Specific Phobia |
| 300.23 | Social Phobia |
| 300.3 | Obsessive-Compulsive Disorder |
| 309.81 | Posttraumatic Stress Disorder |
| 308.3 | Acute Stress Disorder |
| 300.02 | Generalized Anxiety Disorder |

## EATING DISORDERS

| | |
|---|---|
| 307.1 | Anorexia Nervosa |
| 307.51 | Bulimia Nervosa |

307.50    Eating Disorder NOS

## ADJUSTMENT DISORDERS
309.xx    Adjustment Disorder
    .0        With Depressed Mood
    .24       With Anxiety
    .28       With Mixed Anxiety and Depressed Mood
    .3        With Disturbance of Conduct
    .4        With Mixed Disturbance of Emotions and Conduct
    .9        Unspecified

## PERSONALITY DISORDERS
301.0     Paranoid Personality Disorder
301.20    Schizoid Personality Disorder
301.22    Schizotypal Personality Disorder
301.7     Antisocial Personality Disorder
301.83    Borderline Personality Disorder
301.50    Histrionic Personality Disorder
301.81    Narcissistic Personality Disorder
301.82    Avoidant Personality Disorder
301.6     Dependent Personality Disorder
301.4     Obsessive-Compulsive Personality Disorder
301.9     Personality Disorder NOS

# Index

# Order Form

**Current Clinical Strategies books can also be purchased at all medical bookstores**

| Title | Book | CD |
|---|---|---|
| Treatment Guidelines in Medicine, 2006 Edition | $19.95 | $36.95 |
| Psychiatry History Taking, Third Edition | $12.95 | $28.95 |
| Psychiatry, 2008 Edition | $12.95 | $28.95 |
| Pediatric Drug Reference, 2004 Edition | $9.95 | $28.95 |
| Anesthesiology, 2008 Edition | $16.95 | $28.95 |
| Medicine, 2007 Edition | $16.95 | $28.95 |
| Pediatric Treatment Guidelines, 2007 Edition | $19.95 | $29.95 |
| Physician's Drug Manual, 2005 Edition | $9.95 | $28.95 |
| Surgery, Sixth Edition | $12.95 | $28.95 |
| Gynecology and Obstetrics, 2008 Edition | $16.95 | $30.95 |
| Pediatrics, 2007 Edition | $12.95 | $28.95 |
| Family Medicine, 2008 Edition | $26.95 | $46.95 |
| History and Physical Examination in Medicine, Tenth Edition | $14.95 | $28.95 |
| Outpatient and Primary Care Medicine, 2008 Edition | $16.95 | $28.95 |
| Critical Care Medicine, 2007 Edition | $16.95 | $32.95 |
| Handbook of Psychiatric Drugs, 2008 Edition | $14.95 | $28.95 |
| Pediatric History and Physical Examination, Fourth Edition | $12.95 | $28.95 |
| Current Clinical Strategies CD-ROM Collection for Palm, Pocket PC, Windows, and Macintosh | | $49.95 |

CD-ROMs are compatible with Palm, Pocket PC, Windows and Macintosh.

| Quantity | Title | Amount |
|---|---|---|
|  |  |  |
|  |  |  |
|  |  |  |
|  |  |  |
|  |  |  |

**Order by Phone:** 800-331-8227 or 949-348-8404
**Fax:** 800-965-9420 or 949-348-8405
**Internet Orders:** http://www.ccspublishing.com/ccs
**Mail Orders:**

Current Clinical Strategies Publishing
PO Box 1753
Blue Jay, CA 92317

C r e d i t     C a r d     N u m b e r :
_____

**Exp:** ___/___

A shipping charge of $5.00 will be added to each order

**Signature:** _____

**Phone Number:** (_____)_____

**Name and Address (please print):**

_____

_____

_____

_____